NARCISSISTIC ABUSE RECOVERY

THE POWER TO SURVIVE AND TO ESCAPE FROM THE COVERT AND EMOTIONAL ABUSE OF A NARCISSIST TOXIC RELATIONSHIP. A SURVIVAL GUIDE TO UNDERSTANDING WHEN TO GO AWAY OR STAY

HOPE UTARAM

Table of Contents

Introduction

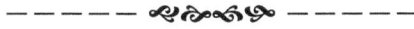

————— ❧❦❧❦ —————

Unless you live under a rock you've definitely heard the word narcissism. In fact, the World Narcissistic Abuse Awareness day, usually celebrated on the first of June, clearly shows that the world acknowledges narcissism to a high degree. Due to the increased spread of information among the public from every corner, the meaning of narcissism has become so diluted such that even harmless people are labeled narcissists based on what they share on social media.

It is ironical that despite the popularity of the word, only a small percentage of the population understands what narcissistic abuse really is. Lambe et al. (2018) in analyzing how narcissism leads to violence and aggression, define narcissistic abuse as a form of psychological and emotional torture which is inflicted by people associated with a lack of conscience and who have antisocial disorders. Narcissism is the condition where one possesses an inflated sense of themselves. A narcissist seeks gratification from their unrealistic self-image hence they have trouble maintaining relationships. The same love and attention that they seek from others, they are unable to reciprocate. They lack empathy and have troubled relationships. Their idealized self-image covers a great vulnerability that is sensitive to the slightest criticism. Narcissism develops from a troubled childhood exposed to traumas, in which one feels unloved and develops a deep sense of inferiority. Therefore, narcissists seek validation from the people they identify as the most appropriate targets who will worship at their feet. They disguise their hidden motives with love for the would-be victim and after trapping them, they manipulate them to fulfill their selfish motives. Narcissism is real, and it has wounded various people in society. People who had their life together become off course and if one is not careful, they end up in great harm.

It is difficult to comprehend how someone professes to love you then goes right ahead to abuse you, but the truth is, love and loyalty do not always exist together. In an era where various people find their partners from social networking sites, it is easy to find yourself under the embrace of a narcissist because you can hardly assess their background or anyone else, they have dated in the past. Online matchmaking businesses are on the rise and anyone not in a relationship seems interested. Those who want to love and be loved are being targeted by these businesses ready to hook everyone up with "like-minded" individuals. First, this boom of the business shows that people are increasingly and desperately looking for love. Second, it has greatly increased the risk of encountering imperfect matches.

This book aims at showing you how you can fully recover from the abuse of a narcissist and resume your original self. It equips you with the knowledge to understand when you are in a relationship with a narcissist and how to end it. Notwithstanding, you will be able to help other people you know who might be in such abusive situations. It brings to you the good news that most narcissists are predictable, and you can use their vulnerabilities to your advantage.

Chapter 1

─ ─ ─ ─ ─ ❧❦❧❦ ─ ─ ─ ─ ─

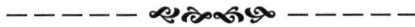

Defining Narcissistic Behavior in Simple Terms

Understanding how narcissists think and who they are most likely to target for narcissistic abuse, you are now in a much better position to deal with any narcissists in your life. Whether the narcissist in question is a spouse, romantic partner, family member, friend, or boss, these tips and strategies will help you keep a clear head and respond effectively.

Effective Responses

There are a number of effective responses to narcissistic abuse, but they all have one thing in common: an understanding of what the narcissist really wants. No matter what seems to be happening at the moment, the narcissist is always looking for power. The most effective responses are those which allow you to keep your power rather than giving any more of it away to the narcissist. This means not allowing the narcissist to disregard your boundaries, but it also means not reacting emotionally in ways that might make the narcissist more powerful in the situation.

Clarify Your Boundaries

The first and most important step is to clarify your boundaries. For a codependent person, developing clear boundaries is always difficult. One of the defining characteristics of codependency is a lack of clarity about where the self ends and where others begin, so you may need to clarify that for yourself before you can begin to establish boundaries with the other people in your life. You are not responsible for how other people feel, for what they do, or for the consequences of their actions. You are only ever responsible for your own actions.

To start the process, make a list describing how you want to be treated by the other people in your life. The list should have clear statements about the kind of behavior you aren't willing to tolerate. For example, "no putting me down" or "no guilt-tripping."

Making a list might be a little challenging, especially if your self-esteem is badly damaged or if you've been conditioned to feel that you don't have any rights. If you feel like you're always responsible for other people's emotional reactions, you might feel guilty about setting boundaries.

If this is how you're feeling, remind yourself that you have the same rights as anyone else. First and foremost, you have the right to say, "no." One way to write your list of boundaries is to ask yourself what you wish you could say "no" to. Everything you wish you could say "no" to is a boundary you can set.

For instance, if your mother always calls you on the weekend and asks you to run errands for her no matter what else you had planned, you probably wish you could say no in that situation. The truth is that you can—you just need to establish a clear boundary. Add "not doing errands for Mom without advance notice" to your list of boundaries.

Once you have your list, attach a realistic consequence to each boundary. For example, "if anyone tries to make me feel guilty, I will not do what they are asking me to do," or "if anyone shouts at me, I will leave and go someplace safe."

The consequences should not be retaliation, just basic and logical steps to protect yourself and your own boundaries. For every situation in your life that feels abusive or manipulative, you should have a clearly-defined boundary and a clearly-defined consequence. The goal is to know just what you will do ahead of time, so you don't need to react emotionally when the situation comes up.

Assert Yourself

Asserting yourself is not the same as being aggressive or hostile and is completely different from being passive-aggressive or resentful. In order to assert yourself effectively, it's essential to stay calm. Stand up for yourself but don't let the narcissist push your buttons. He will almost certainly try!

Be as direct as possible. For example, if your partner launches into a tirade about your shortcomings, don't respond with a counterattack or a resentful hint about how you're feeling. Instead, just tell them that you aren't willing to participate in a conversation where you're being put down, then walk away from the conversation.

If someone is trying to guilt-trip you into spending time with them, tell them you aren't available and leave it at that. If they tell you that you don't care about them because of the boundary you're setting, tell them you disagree, or you see it differently.

Whenever you assert yourself, be as clear as possible about what you are willing to do and what you aren't willing to do. Stick to the boundaries you've set and refuse to engage with any attempts to manipulate you.

If the person you're talking to is being abusive, confront what they're doing in the clearest terms. For example, "I don't like it when you call me stupid. If you want to continue this conversation, don't do that again."

To establish clear boundaries may take a little while because the narcissist has to see that you really mean it. He will try to push it, testing to see if your resolve will weaken. Follow through with your consequences every single time, and the narcissist will either learn to respect them or leave the situation.

Projection

Projection is simple if an immature psychological defense mechanism in which negative emotions and self-criticism are projected outward onto another person to avoid having to face them directly. Narcissists use projection all the time because their true or inner self is the complete opposite from the false or ideal self they want others to see.

Whenever anything reminds them of how they really feel inside, they defend themselves by projecting the negative emotion onto another person. When the narcissist is feeling incompetent, he will accuse you of incompetence. When the narcissist is feeling ugly, he will call you ugly. When the narcissist is feeling worthless and unlovable, he will do everything in his power to make you feel worthless and unlovable.

Understanding this process is the key to not being controlled by it. If you have unclear boundaries, it's hard not to absorb what the narcissist is saying. When your boundaries are stronger, you can see that the narcissist isn't really talking about you at all—she's talking about how she feels inside.

You can deal with sniping and minor put-downs by refusing to react the way the narcissist is hoping for. The narcissist is always looking for an emotional response because no matter what the emotion is, it demonstrates the power the narcissist holds in the situation. If you respond calmly and don't take the bait, you can avoid giving them any more power. For example, if your partner says, "the house is a terrible mess, you never do anything around here," you can say, "yes, it could stand to be picked up, should we do that now?" without reacting to the accusation.

It's sometimes better to ignore anything hinted or implied but to respond directly to insults or put-downs by setting a firm boundary. Either way, the key point is to not react in any way that will give the narcissist more of the power he craves.

Remind yourself that he isn't really talking about you in the first place. He's really describing his own inner self—the self that he can't stand to face or deal with. Don't take it personally, but don't let him use it as an excuse to mistreat you. The narcissist's actions may be driven by suffering, but he has no right to inflict suffering on you as his coping strategy.

Codependency often makes it difficult to deal with projection because the codependent person also has a painful relationship with the inner self. You may have received toxic messages in childhood that gave you a distorted sense of who you are. For instance, you may have such a negative self-picture that you find it easy to accept criticism and almost impossible to accept praise. When someone tells you something good about yourself, you can't hear or it or believe it. When someone tells you something bad about yourself, it feels like the truth.

Your negative self-image comes from your own experiences and has nothing to do with whatever criticism or blame the narcissist is throwing at you. It might feel like he sees the horrible truth about you, but that really isn't what's happening at all. The narcissist cannot see the inner you, for good or bad, so his comments can never represent some special insight into who you really are. No matter what terrible thing he says, he's always describing how he feels about himself. It's always a projection.

It's important to work on your self-esteem, which may mean getting therapy to deal with the toxic beliefs you absorbed in childhood. Whether you're in therapy or not, understanding projection is essential in dealing with narcissistic abuse.

Dealing with Narcissistic Parents

For many people with codependency, the first narcissist they ever met was their mother or father. Establishing boundaries can be much harder with family than with other people because family usually knows you a lot better and has a lot more practice pushing your buttons.

Some people choose not to deal with their parents at all because they can't establish boundaries in any other way. If you still want to maintain a relationship with your parents, learning how to have better boundaries may be the only way to do it.

The key is to detach, which doesn't mean to move far away (although that works for some people) or to stop caring but to stop taking on the responsibility for your parent's feelings. Just because your mother wants something does not mean it is your responsibility to provide it. Just because your father expects you to prioritize him at all times doesn't mean you have to.

For example, if your mother expects you to take her phone calls even when you're busy, you may feel like a bad child if you don't take the call. However, you're not responsible for managing her emotions. Take a step back and detach emotionally, then tell her you'll call her when you're no longer busy. That doesn't make you a bad child—it just means you have to manage your time like everyone else.

Your mother or father may try to guilt-trip you for not going along with what they want. For instance, they may send you texts or leave voice mail messages to blackmail you emotionally. Set clear boundaries when this happens: "If you want me to spend more time with you, I need you to stop sending me this kind of message."

Some people find it easier to establish healthy boundaries when they can keep a little more distance between themselves and their family members. For instance, it might help to stay with friends or at an Airbnb when you're visiting home, rather than to sleep at your parents' house. This allows you to take a little space when you need to withdraw while still spending time with your family.

Ineffective Responses

Some tactics are effective when dealing with a narcissist, and some are ineffective. Remember to avoid these common but ineffective responses, especially if you have a history of codependency:

- Placating the narcissist

- Arguing with the narcissist

- Defending your own actions

- Criticizing the narcissist

- Begging or pleading

- Blaming yourself

- Making empty threats

- Excusing, minimizing, or denying the problem

- Avoiding conflict

- Trying to get the narcissist to understand you

Don't Placate

Placating the narcissist will only backfire because he will interpret your attempts to appease him as a victory. Narcissists see interpersonal conflict in black and white terms—every disagreement has a winner and a loser. If you appease the narcissist, he will only take this as an admission of defeat, encouraging him to continue with the same behaviors. Once you draw a line with a narcissist, you have to stick to that line.

Don't Argue

Arguing back and forth with a narcissist is a lose-lose proposition because it's based on the false assumption that the narcissist shares your desire for eventual agreement and mutual understanding. In reality, the narcissist only cares about who wins and who loses. Facts are irrelevant to the narcissist, so debating things like who said what or who did what can only play into the narcissist's hands. Deflect every attempt to draw you into a debate. The narcissist isn't arguing in good faith anyway, so trying to win an argument or prove your point would only waste your time and energy.

Don't Defend

It's only natural to defend your actions or your motivations when someone is criticizing you, but defending yourself is always a mistake when you're dealing with a narcissist. Why? It's because the narcissist is assuming something that she doesn't have any right to assume, which is that she has the authority to judge your actions as acceptable or unacceptable. The same thing goes for explaining yourself, which tells the narcissist that she has the right to demand explanations. As an independent person, you have the right to make your own decisions. You don't have to defend or explain yourself to anyone.

Don't Criticize

Criticizing the narcissist is a mistake for several different reasons. First, it assumes that the narcissist actually cares about doing the right thing, when in reality, he only cares about getting his own needs met. Second, it opens you up to the narcissist's counterattack—after all, if you can judge him, then he can judge you. Third, it can trigger an explosive burst of narcissistic rage. Narcissists cannot handle even a hint of criticism because it exposes the vulnerability and pain of the inner self. Rather than criticizing the narcissist for his selfish actions, it's better to establish and enforce your own boundaries.

Don't Beg

In the black-and-white mental world of the typical narcissist, those who beg and plead are weak and contemptible, while those who receive these pleas are strong and powerful. When you plead with a narcissist to change his behavior, he sees this as a clear confirmation that he is strong and you are weak. Instead of doing whatever you're begging him to do, the narcissist will simply view you with even more contempt and disregard. It can be hard to remember this, but you are only ever in control of your own actions. Focus on what you can do —not on what he should do.

Don't Blame Yourself

If you cannot control the narcissist's actions (and you really can't), then you cannot be responsible for them either. The only person responsible for any action is the person who commits that action. When the narcissist yells or gets drunk or punches holes in the walls, those actions are his and his alone. It's impossible for you to provoke them or bear any responsibility for them whatsoever. Remember, codependent people have a hard time understanding and establishing boundaries between themselves and others. It may feel like you are somehow to blame for what the narcissist says or does or feels, but you are two separate people and can only be responsible for your own life.

Don't Bluff

Don't ever make a threat you aren't prepared to carry out because the narcissist will take this as a sign that you don't really mean it and that he can ignore any boundaries you try to set. For example, don't say "if I catch you cheating again, I'll move out" unless you fully intend to do exactly that.

Don't Deny It

Denial is one of the strongest instincts the codependent person has, and you'll have to fight against it for a long time if that's part of your history and your personality. When you know something isn't right, it won't help at all to pretend otherwise. It's better to face it and get it dealt with, even if you find that painful or difficult. This includes making excuses for the narcissist's behavior or minimizing how bad the problem really is.

Don't Avoid It

Avoiding a problem is a lot like denying it and will do nothing in the long term to regain your power over your own life. Fleeing the scene of a conversation you have lost control over may sometimes be necessary so you can get your emotions under control and stop playing whatever game the narcissist wants you to play. However, you can't establish boundaries by simply avoiding any conflict, so in the end, you will have to address the situation one way or the other.

Don't Look for Sympathy or Understanding

Trying to get the narcissist to understand where you're coming from or even to sympathize with you is a losing fight. The narcissist isn't interested in understanding other people, only in getting what he needs from them. He may express sympathy under certain conditions, but his ability to actually feel it is limited or nonexistent. The goal in dealing with a narcissist is not to be understood, but to establish boundaries and make sure they're respected.

Dealing with Physical Abuse

Physical abuse is not always the most psychologically damaging form of abuse. Many people find that emotional abuse is more harmful to their overall wellbeing. However, physical abuse is dangerous in a different way because it almost always escalates over time. Many abusers will express intense shame and remorse over their violent acts in the immediate aftermath, but that doesn't mean they won't do it again. They almost certainly will, no matter what they say— and it will almost certainly get worse.

The abuser may try to evade the responsibility for their own violence by blaming it on you, so boundaries are especially important in this type of situation. You can't be responsible for the other person's actions, so if they say you provoked them or drove them to it, they are simply trying to dodge responsibility. It is never your fault.

If your partner is physically abusive, threatening, or violent, it's important not to minimize the problem. Denial can literally be deadly. Seek help immediately and make a plan to ensure your own safety. No matter how strongly you feel about the other person, don't kid yourself about a violent relationship. It's never acceptable for anyone to hit you, and if you don't take steps immediately, it will happen again.

Chapter 2

────── ❧❦❧❦ ──────

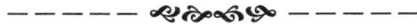

Overcoming Negative Personality Traits

There are several different tactics that narcissists use to manipulate and abuse other people. The list that will be used in this chapter is not comprehensive, by any means, but it does cover the most commonly used tactics that narcissists employ. Each of these manipulation tactics can be harmful in their own ways, and each is meant to keep you in line for the narcissist, doing whatever it is that the narcissist wants you to do, and providing him with a steady stream of narcissistic supply.

The False Self

As briefly touched upon earlier, the narcissist creates a false self in an attempt to manipulate others into liking him. The false self is used to draw people in and is constantly changing. Perhaps one of the most unnerving things about watching a narcissist from a distance is watching him change as he goes from person to person. He may have certain quirks and mannerisms with one person, but then as soon as he moves to the next, his mannerisms change completely. This is because he is constantly mirroring their mannerisms in an attempt to get them to like them more.

Remember, people like those they relate to, and one of the easiest ways to build rapport or a relationship between people is through mirroring. People naturally mirror people that they like or are close to. You can see this if you watch a couple at a restaurant for a date. You may see them choose to take a sip of their drinks at the same time, or both prop themselves up on their elbows as they talk. This is because they are in sync. If you had the ability to view their breathing and heart rates, you would likely be met with the surprise that they are both quite similar as well. The narcissist preys off of this way of synchronizing with others, using it to his advantage to create bonds where none would naturally develop. It is perhaps the closest thing to empathy that the narcissist is capable of.

The false self serves another purpose as well—the narcissist uses it as a shield between his fragile inner sense of self and the world around him. He pretends to be someone more confident, so people do not realize the truth about him. He uses it to be charismatic, in hopes of drawing more victims near, or in order to develop enough of a positive reputation that there is no way for his victim to leave and actually get anyone to believe that the narcissist was abusive.

This goes one step further and allows the narcissist to feel better about himself as well. He feels more comfortable and confident in the skin of another because he, himself, has a very fragile, fractured sense of self. The person he is inside is not one to be proud of, and he is aware of that. When he takes on the persona of someone else, however, he is able to better live with himself. He acts as if he is another person, and he gets valuable information from this. He learns what works and what does not, which traits are more and less desirable, and more. By learning this information, he is better able to manipulate others in the future. He knows how to tweak his behaviors by watching the people he emulates and how they manage to get through the world. This makes him more effective in general.

Idealization-Devaluation-Discard Cycle

The idealization-devaluation-discard cycle is the cycle in which the narcissist puts you onto a pedestal and then knocks you off of it just as quickly, leaving you reeling and unsure of your place in his life. It is used to manipulate and hook you onto the narcissist, where he will keep you until he has decided you have done your job and he is bored with you.

Idealization

The first stage, idealization, involves what is referred to as love bombs. This stage seeks to build you up, showering you with love and affection. The narcissist pushes for the relationship to move quicker than you may be comfortable, and comes onto you with more tenacity than is typically expected early in a relationship. He wants you to feel the most intense whirlwind romance you have ever felt, and he mirrors exactly the person you want him to be. The persona he creates is everything you have ever desired at this stage, and he will show you how loving and affectionate he can be.

At this stage, he is listening closely to everything you say, learning all about you and your insecurities. Any information you provide at this stage when you are confiding in someone that you think you can trust, can, and will, be used against you later on. The narcissist will be attentive now, but it is only to learn what he can use to manipulate you when the time comes.

The idealization stage continues to pick up the pace over time, and the narcissist grows more clingy and affectionate. He always wants to spend time with you, and you quickly explain this away as passion or try to perceive his overzealousness as romance. You quickly find yourself hooked to the intensity, enjoying every moment of it, and you eventually want to seek it out yourself. You find yourself just as willing to spend time with the narcissist as he is to spend time with you, and your relationship with him slowly begins to consume other aspects of your life. You start spending more and more time with the narcissist and less time with others around you.

Devaluation

Just as quickly as the spark in your relationship caught fire, you quickly find it burning away. The narcissist seems to be pulling away at this stage, and you cannot figure out why. If you ask what is wrong, the narcissist denies there is a problem at all. He insists that everything is fine, but the distance has been put between you. He may begin to demean you or call you names, implying that you are wrong about things, or that you are unworthy of his time.

Confused, you find yourself desperate to figure out what changed so suddenly. You do not understand why the narcissist suddenly withdrew affection from you and replaced it with this. The reason for it is he has decided to devalue you. The purpose of this is to get you yearning for more. You do whatever it takes to get back into the narcissist's good graces, knowing that is where you want to be. You want to be with the narcissist when he is loving, not when he sees you as invaluable. He takes advantage of this and realizes that you have, effectively, been ensnared into his web and you will be willing to put up with his mistreatment. He may move back to the idealize stage at this point if you have done a sufficient job of proving that you are willing to do whatever it takes to keep him happy, or he may move on to the discard stage.

Discard

Eventually, the narcissist decides that he no longer wants you around. Maybe you were not willing enough to put up with his abuse, or maybe he has found someone else that puts up with it better. Narcissists prefer not to work much for what they want and will often take the path of least resistance to getting their narcissistic supply. If you are no longer the path of least resistance, you will be discarded.

At this point, the narcissist essentially cuts you off. He likely will not respond to messages you send or your attempts to reconcile with him. He instead moves on just as quickly as he flew into your life, ready to move on to other victims.

Sometimes, the narcissist will eventually move back from discarding you to idealizing you again. This may happen if he decides that he wants to keep you around as a backup, or maybe he has decided he wants something you have to offer that other people do not. Regardless of the reason, the cycle will begin again at this point, starting with idealizing.

Gaslighting

Gaslighting is one of the most dangerous manipulation tactics narcissists use. This one involves the narcissist convincing you that you are crazy or incapable of understanding the reality around you. When the narcissist decides to gaslight you, he wants you to discount your own perception of what happened and instead focus on the one he insists happened. Of course, the narcissist is trying to instill a false narrative into you rather than the truth.

He does this over time to weaken your perceived grasp on reality. If you are questioned repeatedly on whether your memory is faulty or not, you are prone to believing it eventually, especially when it comes from someone you love and trust not to hurt you. This is what makes this abuse so insidious—the victim has trusted the abuser, and it has been betrayed so thoroughly that the victim feels as though he or she can no longer trust reality as he or she perceives it.

The narcissist most frequently does this through denying your account of what happened. If you say that the narcissist started a fight, he will either vehemently deny that a fight happened at all, saying you must have imagined it and asking if you are okay, or he will say that you did something to instigate it rather than allowing the blame to remain on him. Either way, the perception of the truth has been altered in some way, and the narcissist is counting on you trusting the narcissist enough to disbelieve yourself rather than disbelieving the narcissist. After all, most people would not think that someone would attempt to make them think they are insane, especially if it is someone they think loves them.

Frequently, the declarations of something being false or having never happened will be matched with the narcissist pointing out some other times where you really did forget something. If you forgot all about an appointment you had last week, for example, the narcissist might point that out and then look at you in concern and ask if you are doing okay. He may imply that you need to see a psychologist, or that you seem to be losing touch with reality, which is terrifying to most people. You are then left feeling doubtful about what had really happened. Rather than speaking your mind about it, you instead nod your head and agree with the narcissist, not wanting to push the point or come across as crazy. To people who are not abusive, the idea of playing with someone's mind in this manner is absolutely abhorrent, so you do not think that the narcissist may be manipulating you, particularly if you do not know what the narcissist is at this point.

The ultimate irony here, however, is that the narcissist is the one with the skewed perception of reality. In fact, he may have even gaslit himself to believe what he is convincing you of, and that is what makes him so credible—he may literally believe what he is saying if it fits his narrative better than what actually happened. Ultimately, when in doubt, you should trust your gut. Especially if you have been wondering if you are being abused, you should never trust what the narcissist may be saying to you. Your own perception

Smear Campaigns

Smear campaigns involve the narcissist attempting to absolutely destroy another's reputation through any means possible. The ultimate goal is to entirely and irrevocably tarnish someone's image that they feel as though they have been cast out of their social circles. This most typically happens when you have somehow enraged a narcissist in one way or another, and the narcissist feels the need to seek revenge on you and make sure that you are ultimately the more injured party.

Imagine that you have just cut off your narcissistic ex after finally divorcing. The narcissist, feeling as though he cannot possibly allow someone to tarnish his own image through cutting him off, he instead creates a story in which he has actually divorced and cut you off. Usually, his reason for having done so is one that most people would find absolutely abhorrent, and it may even be the reason you have chosen to divorce him. For example, if you divorced him because he cheated on you in your own home, going so far as to bring the other women into your own bed, that you, personally bought, and then he proceeded to attack you or physically assaulted you after you confronted him, he would spin that story around to everyone else instead. You would be the one having an affair in his bed, and you had attacked him when he walked in and started crying because he ruined the mood.

The narcissist would then spin this tale to everyone who would listen. If you live in a small town, he will tell everyone: The grocer, the gas station attendant, and even random people he passes walking his dog. The point is to ruin your image, and he holds nothing back. He even spins things around to say that he is such a great person for not pressing charges because he just loves you so much and wants the best for you, even if the best is not him.

The lies may not stop there and include stories about how you had been on drugs, or that you stole a car when drunk one night and that you gave him several STIs. He will stop at nothing to destroy your reputation in order to protect his own and damage yours.

He will insist on all of this so adamantly that some people are likely to believe him, and that can be the end to you being able to find work in a small town, where reputation is everything. At the end of the day, the narcissist does this to regain control of a situation that spiraled out of his control. You may have cut him off, but he got the final word in by ruining your hometown for you. You can either deal with the rumors and attempting damage control, or you can move on with your life and hope that the narcissist does not find you again.

Remember, even though the narcissist has flung this at you, you can be the better person and choose not to engage at all. You will probably be happier in the long run if you refuse to confront him about his lies. All that would do is prove to him that he could get a reaction out of you, and he will remember that tactic for future use.

Triangulation

Triangulation involves three people who are interacting with each other, in which one attempts to manipulate, deceive, and abuse another person through weaponizing a third person. It involves three different people: the persecutor, the rescuer, and the persecuted.

The persecutor is someone who believes that he has been victimized in some way, shape, or form. He feels as though he has been hurt somehow, though his internalized victim role is most likely unjustified in this instance. As you have learned, the narcissist thrives on victimizing himself, even when he has been the one that hurt other people.

Typically, the triangle begins when the narcissist wrongs the persecuted, who responds unfavorably. The persecuted may call him out for such egregious behavior and request not to be disrespected again. Even though the persecuted could have said that in the nicest way possible, with a smile on his face and offering the narcissist a friendship bouquet, the narcissist takes some sort of fault with what has been said. He feels ashamed that he was called out, and he uses that shame to say he is the victim.

The narcissist then calls out to the rescuer to come to his aid. He does not see any issue using someone else to fight his battles, as the ends justify the means every time for the narcissist. The narcissist tells the rescuer some sort of lie about what has happened, skewing it just enough so that the story is compelling enough for the rescuer to get involved. He may say that the persecuted has been talking badly about both the persecutor and the rescuer, or he may say that the persecuted has been intending to take advantage of you both. No matter what he says, it is fabricated in order to get the rescuer to also seek to discontinue a relationship with the persecuted.

The persecuted, much as the person who was a victim to a smear campaign, finds his reputation completely destroyed and may have even lost a relationship or job due to the narcissist's actions. Meanwhile, the narcissist happily sits in his corner, content that his own vigilante justice has been served. He does not care about the implications of his actions, or that the persecuted if he has lost a job due to the narcissist's behaviors, can continue to feed his family. The narcissist does not care about anyone involved beyond himself.

The persecuted is then left trying to pick up the pieces of his life that are left behind, particularly if the consequences of the triangulation were devastating, and trying to move on with life. The narcissist is then able to get away with this behavior, despite how unfair it was, and how wrong the narcissist's behaviors were. He can try to defend himself, but he is likely only going to be the victim of a further attack from the narcissist and the narcissist's rescuer in response.

Chapter 3

------ ✥❧❦✥ ------

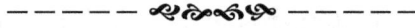

Understanding Your Thinking

How that you have learned about the healing process and how spiritual healing works, it is time to move onto the next aspect of healing.

Just like a house that has four walls, you are also made up of four walls. These four walls or pillars are what make you the person you are and help you in creating an identity for yourself.

The four pillars are as follows:

- self-esteem

- self-worth

- self-trust

- self-love

You must have noticed that throughout the book, these words have been used generously. These are the four pillars on which every human being stands. These pillars offer the support to live life, to tackle problems that life throws at you and to finally experience a fulfilled life.

Relationship with a narcissist hurts so much and causes internal damage because a narcissist methodically attacks all the four pillars. He ensures that he leaves no stone unturned in damaging every small part of all the four pillars leaving no option for you other than to fall.

To help you understand this better, imagine a storm that is raging through. Have you ever seen the destruction a storm causes and have you wondered how long it takes for the people and homes affected by the storm to reclaim their life back?

You are exactly similar to the person caught in a storm. A narcissist attacks you unannounced just like a storm when you least expect it or are least prepared. He attacks all your pillars and disturbs the foundation on which you are standing, so you fall and collapse just like those houses that fall in a storm or massive trees that get uprooted. The destruction is so much that it takes months and in some cases years for the pillars to rebuild.

There are some basic practices that you can do to help rebuild the pillars.

Self-Esteem

Self-esteem essentially means supporting yourself. It is how much control you have over yourself, your mind, your body, and your behaviors. Self-esteem is also about the perception you have about yourself and how you see yourself.

The opposite of self-esteem is self-sabotage or self-damage. During the process of healing, it is important that you build your self-esteem.

You can begin by doing simple things that will tell you that you are in control of the situation. You can start by tackling basic things such as hygiene that you might be ignoring right now because of your PTSD or depression. Something as simple as having a daily routine to take a shower or to dress decently even when at home can help you regain a sense of control. These baby steps will help you tackle the bigger problems.

Self-Worth

This is about knowing your value and respecting your worth. It is believing that you are worth the respect, love, and affection. The exact opposite of self-worth is shame and unworthiness.

After the abuse, the narcissist would have ensured that you feel a deep sense of shame and hate yourself. Self-worth is also about speaking up for your rights and standing up for yourself and what you believe in.

You need to focus on the courage to build self-worth. Courage does not mean trying to scale the mountains or running in the wild. Courage means taking measures to change your life actively. It can be applying for another job, being able to negotiate a good pay that you deserve, applying to school if you always wanted to finish school, etc. It means identifying something that you wanted to do but have never done because you believed that you were not worth it.

It also comes by not compromising on your values or doing things you are uncomfortable doing. You would have compromised on your values while trying to appease the narcissist. Once you develop courage, you will not compromise on your values and thus will develop self-worth. Regardless of what you have come to believe about yourself, God our father has a very different view of who you are. I choose to believe that his word and it changed my life completely. I went from feeling lost, to finding hope in his promises. If you haven't read that book yet, I suggest you do. If you have tried everything else, and years after leaving your abuser you still feel stuck, angry, and broken, I suggest you start by getting a bible. Read as frequently as possible and I guarantee you would see a change in your life.

Self-Trust

Self-trust is about trusting yourself, your judgment. It means having faith in yourself and being confident about your decisions. It means not second guessing every single decision and worrying about it.

When you lack self-trust, you live in constant fear and doubt. During the relationship with the narcissist, you slowly start losing self-trust without even you realizing. It happens silently, and before you know it, you will be second-guessing everything. The narcissist achieves this by gaslighting and deflecting blame.

The only way to rebuild self-trust is to listen to your intuition. The gut feeling that everyone talks about is what you must pay attention to. If something does not feel right to you, then trust that instinct and let it go. Gut feeling is more tangible than some more forms of intuition. Gut feeling is never wrong, as it is your inner voice trying to guide you and protect you from danger or from something that is not right for you.

Your gut feeling and intuition stop working once you start ignoring them. It is like ignoring your best friend who has nothing but the best intentions for you. Once you start ignoring your intuition and gut, they no longer guide you, and that is when you take the wrong steps.

Get it back by listening to it. Follow whatever your gut says and see the change.

Self-Love

Finally, the fourth pillar, self-love is about caring and nurturing yourself. It is about treating yourself well. Self-love takes a back seat during the relationship with a narcissist because the narcissist wants and demands all the love. When you are in a relationship with a narcissist, you cease to be in a relationship with yourself. You slowly stop loving yourself and go into self-denial and self-judgment mode. You judge yourself poorly and try to rationalize all the bad behavior being shown by the narcissist. When you do not love yourself, you go into a people-pleasing mode and develop a savior complex. By now, you know how dangerous savior complex is to your health and sanity. You start believing you are ugly and stop taking care of your health.

The medicine to this lies in loving yourself back. This can be accomplished by taking small steps such as cooking your favorite meal, eating healthy food, and eating regular meals. It could also be treating yourself at a salon or spa and just pampering yourself.

You can focus on things that you want to change about yourself and more importantly accept what you cannot change. Self-acceptance is a part of self-love because if you do not accept yourself just as you are, then there is no way that another person or the world will accept you the way you are. This is because others will treat you just as well or as bad as you treat yourself. By treating yourself well, you are teaching the world how they must treat you and conveying your boundaries and wishes to them.

How Long Does It Take to Heal Completely?

This is a question that haunts most victims because it can seem like forever with no end in sight. A lot of days you may go to bed wishing that you do not have to get up the next morning because you are afraid how bad the day will be. You will constantly feel like there is no light at the end of the tunnel.

Do not drown in this hopelessness because this kind of negative thinking will quickly take you back to victim land. The journey to victim land is a free airplane ride where you will reach the deepest levels of fear, hatred, and disgust within minutes, but remember that journey to victim land means no return.

Hence, hold onto your horses. Take comfort in the fact that God has given you this amazing opportunity to heal you, and you can start by drawing closer to him. Healing that comes from your spirit, is exactly what you need for psychological abuse, just because a lot of the scars you have are not physical ones.

There are countless women who spend their entire lives trapped in victim land and never live a happy and fulfilled life.

The truth is that there is no timeline for healing. It is not a mathematical calculation with definite results. Do not trust anyone who is telling you that it takes no more than a month or two to recover. Neither must you pay attention to fellow victims who claim to have healed in record time. You are not in competition with anyone, this is about the rest of your life, and healing needs to be thorough and deep to be sustainable.

This journey is a spiritual journey, and the destination is you, so it can be one month for some; it can take one year for some, and some people can take several years. Healing depends on various factors, but above all, it depends on how committed you are to the process. At times you will see no progress at all. There will also be times when from one forward stage you will take two steps back for reasons you cannot understand yourself. Despite this, persist. Persistence works magic. Keep a journal and write down everything so that when you feel demotivated, you can turn back the pages and see how far you have come.

Celebrate each milestone and make a note of it. Acknowledgment helps develop self-love and will bring you to acceptance. Again, you need to understand that you are not in competition with anyone but yourself in this and this not a race. Healing from narcissistic abuse is not like running a sprint, but it is more like a marathon. Hence, pace yourself and keep the momentum going.

It does not matter whether it takes a few months longer, but it is important that you heal completely and come out of the marathon with flying colors.

Chapter 4

------ ❧❦❧ ------

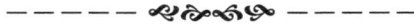

Choices and Self Discovery

When adults mistreated by their abusers begin to develop a positive feeling towards people abusing them, it's referred to as Stockholm syndrome. As the whole abusive situation progresses, you find yourself being childlike and overly reliant on your abuser. You start becoming grateful for even the smallest sign of affection and approval they show you. Eventually, you end up bonding with your captors and end up loving them more.

But again, how do all these apply to a narcissistic relationship?

Stage 1: Continuous rewards with nothing given in return

At the very beginning, the one thing that you have to notice is that your narcissistic individual targets on getting hold of you. That is why they will start giving you emotional pellets in the form of love, validation and affection, sweet gestures and even praises. They make you believe that you are a wonderful person and this makes you right.

The truth is, you are not alone; we all enjoy getting stroked and loved by someone that we like. This is necessarily what we refer to as 'love bombing' all that they are seeking for in return is for you to continue giving them a chance to prove their love for you.

Stage 2: Performance rewards

Once the narcissist feels secure enough with you, they suddenly stop rewarding you continuously. The only thing that you now get is simply positive attention especially when you soothe their ego and do things that make them feel good.

The truth is, you get enough positive attention that you do not realize that now the only time that you get a reward is when you 'press the food bar' so to speak. In other words, the narcissist is grooming you so that you can please them continually in your life.

Stage 3: Increase in devaluation, a decrease in rewards!

During this particular stage, the narcissist starts abusing you and becoming overly critical of you. They want to control you and put you down whatever chance they get even if it means doing it in public. You may get occasional 'rewards,' but the truth is that at this point they are quite unpredictable. The bad stuff is beginning to outweigh the good stuff. In other words, you are now on 'intermittent reinforcement.'

Stage 4: They set you in flames

At this particular point, if you have never been in a narcissistic relationship before, there is a high chance that you will be puzzled by the whole experience wondering how and why this is happening. The answer is with your narcissistic friend who thinks that you are the cause of all the problems. They blame you and think that if you would do a, b, c and stop being 1, 2, 3, everything would be perfect. You end up doubting your perception of reality.

All you can now do at this point is get addicted, leave and hoover. You are addicted to narcissistic validation and approval. The truth is, you have stopped thinking rationally and rather than projecting your hate at the abuser, you become terrified at the thought of losing them to someone else. Due to what we mentioned above about 'trauma bonding' you cannot see the obvious and no longer care how you feel and what damage this is doing to your life.

If you start summoning your inner strength so that you can quit, they suddenly change their tactics. They try all means to make sure that they suck you back in the same way a vacuum cleaner does 'hoover.' They start doing something minor like buying you a small gift, commenting positively on your dressing, linking your social media posts among others. If that does not seem to work, they work harder by simply going back to the 'love bombing' In other words, the more you are resistant, the harder they try to win you back.

At this point, the sad thing is that many of us are vulnerable and we end up getting sucked up into the relationship again. Mostly it is because we start second-guessing whether there is change or if you will end up regretting this decision for the rest of your life and blah blah blah. In other words, what you are doing is ignoring everything that you know about your abuser with the hope that they might have magically transformed into someone more loving, decent, stable and reliable!

The truth is, it is indeed good to feel loved and wanted. But you have to realize that they are just soothing salves for your wounds. Do not forget that they have destroyed you and caused you so much pain yet you invested all your time and resources into the relationship. They did not see that, but they discarded you like trash anyway.

Before you can start making rash decisions and justifying why you are still in the relationship with this narcissist, ask yourself what makes you so sure that they will not do it again and maybe this time, even worse. Just know that, once you get sucked back, they will soon stop rewarding you and the cycle of abuse starts all over again. Understand that narcissist can train even the strongest of people into believing and submitting to them by using the right combination of praise and punishment. Are you ready for that again?

Chapter 5

──────── ❧❦❧❧ ────────

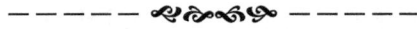

Narcissism in Families

Dealing with a narcissist is incredibly difficult in the best of times, but there are many different ways to manage your relationship. Regardless of whether you are interested in severing all ties for good or you are in a position of having to continue some degree of contact with a narcissist, understanding some of the ways to deal with the narcissist's toxic behaviors can help you minimize your risks of harm and abuse. You can also cause the narcissist to lose interest in you and move on to other targets when you prove yourself invulnerable to his manipulative tactics.

Keep in mind that this will be a trial and error effort, and not every method discussed here may be useful or productive in your unique situation. Consider each method carefully to decide if it meets your needs and can help you, and once you have chosen a method, it is important to remember to keep it up. No matter how much the narcissist may push and try to get your attention back, be consistent in order to get the best effect from your actions. None of these methods are easy, and each will take a gargantuan amount of effort, but when you finally make it to the other side and realize how very free you are from the narcissist's abuse, you will recognize that it was worth every ounce of effort you put into it.

Cutting off the Narcissist

The easiest way to avoid harm from a narcissist is to end the relationship entirely. Refuse to engage in the relationship at all costs. Taking a huge step back from the relationship may be necessary so you can clear your head and see things for what they are. This is typically a permanent change and decision and is the only surefire way to make sure that the narcissistic abuse stops. If you refuse to play the game at all, the narcissist cannot manipulate you.

Furthermore, by refusing any sort of engagement or communication with the narcissist, you are able to deny the narcissist's strongest motivator: Your attention. You suddenly remove yourself as a reliable source of narcissistic supply, and if you continue to deny the narcissist, ultimately, he will have to go elsewhere to meet his need.

Keep in mind that when you do this method, there will be a period that, in psychology, is called an extinction burst. Consider an experiment in which a rat is taught to press a button to get a small nibble of candy. The rat very quickly learns to expect that candy every time the button is pressed, and the behavior of pressing a button becomes positively reinforced. The rat does this to get the candy and does so repeatedly. If the rate goes up and presses the button and one day, it just stops giving out candy, the rat will be confused. It will press the button again and again, with increasing fervor, as it desperately tries to force the button to do what was expected of it and provide more candy. Over time, the rat will lose interest when it becomes clear there is no further reaction, but it will go back to the button occasionally and try to press the button.

Think of the narcissist as the rat and the narcissistic supply as the candy. You are the button to get it. As soon as you cut off contact, the narcissist will suddenly resort to every last strategy that has proven successful in the past in order to try to get your attention and that narcissistic supply desired. He will attempt everything, ranging from love bombs to promises of change and even threats of abuse or suicide if you do not give in. The most important thing to remember is that you cannot give in. No matter what the narcissist says or does, refuse to give him what he wants. His behaviors will escalate more, just like a toddler throwing a fit over having routine broken unexpectedly, and he will not stop at anything that he thinks will be effective. Eventually, however, you will weather the storm, and the narcissist will stop trying. The need for narcissistic supply is too strong, and he will seek it out elsewhere if you continue to refuse. At that point, remember that he will likely come back again in the future to try again, but each attempt will be weaker than the last as he learns that it is useless.

Remember, the period of leaving an abusive relationship is the most dangerous, and the narcissist likely will rely on every physical and emotional threat he can think of. He may threaten to kill himself, you, or other people, or he may begin stalking you. No matter what he does, refuse to engage, and report erratic or dangerous behavior to the appropriate authorities.

Take a Break from the Relationship

Similar to cutting off the narcissist, taking a break from the relationship involves a refusal to communicate. In this case, however, it is not permanent. The break is intended to allow you to clear your head and reevaluate whether you want to continue the relationship. Regardless of what he may accuse you of, remind yourself that this is not a punishment. You did not make this decision to hurt him; you made it protect and care for yourself. You are entitled to controlling who you communicate with, and if you decide that you do not want to talk to the narcissist, you are within your rights to make that choice.

When taking a break from the narcissist, it is appropriate to tell him once that you are taking a break and you will discuss things with him when you are ready. You do not have to provide him with a timeline, no matter how much he may pester you for one, and at that point, you refuse all future contact. You are giving yourself the chance to cool off. You are ensuring that you do not say something that will make the situation worse or inflame the narcissist into doing something harmful.

Do not let the narcissist goad you into responses with accusations of abuse or through playing the victim. You are making a choice that works for you, and ultimately that is the most important part. You need the breathing room and you are taking it. Remind yourself that you owe it to yourself to care for yourself, especially when no one else will. You cannot care for others if you are not caring for yourself.

Healthy Boundaries

Sometimes, cutting off a narcissist is not a viable option, and that is okay. When you have no choice but to continue contact, such as if you are bound by court order to continue a co-parenting relationship, or you work with the narcissist and are not in a position to leave your job, you can focus on mitigating as much harm as possible and protecting yourself from the toxicity the narcissist seems to naturally exude.

Healthy boundaries are one of the easiest techniques to minimize harm from a narcissist, but they are difficult. These boundaries represent a line between what is acceptable and unacceptable to you, and they are to be set at your own prerogative. Boundaries are a healthy part of every relationship, regardless of whether it is a marriage, a friendship, or even with your children. Without boundaries, you will find yourself constantly stepping on toes and breeding resentment.

Unfortunately, narcissists see boundaries as the ultimate insult. It is irresistible to the narcissist, and he will try to stomp on them at every turn. The boundaries set are nothing more than challenges; games to get rises out of you and exert control over your emotional state. When you set these boundaries, you must be prepared to enforce and defend them at all costs.

When the narcissist challenges a boundary, give him one warning. Tell him that if he continues to test your boundary, you will provide a consequence. Tell the narcissist what that consequence for stomping on your boundary is, and every time it is done, you need to enforce the consequence. If you tell the narcissist that you will take an extended break in the event that your boundary is broken, follow through when he stomps on it.

If you tell him you will stop talking to the narcissist if he calls you names in anger and he calls you names, you must immediately disengage and walk away. The key here is to follow through with the entire consequence, no matter how much the narcissist may cry, beg, or threaten.

Disengage

When cutting off is not an option, the next best thing is disengaging emotionally. If you do not invest any emotional energy into your interactions with the narcissist, he will eventually lose interest in you. You can keep your interactions relatively unchanged, but do not pay any attention to the words said, no matter how hurtful they may be. Try to keep in mind that people with NPD are stuck in a developmental stage of a child, unable to feel empathy and wired to be selfish, and remind yourself that if a child had said the things the narcissist spewed at you, you would likely not be very upset or offended at all. After all, children are impulsive, emotional, and irrational. The narcissist hits all three of those traits on the nose, and you should not take the narcissist's actions personally at all.

Disengaging does not mean ignoring or bottling your feelings, however. When you disengage, acknowledge what was said and give it the consideration it deserves, which is, admittedly, very little. This can be particularly difficult if the narcissist is a loved one that you trusted, but remember to try to disregard the emotional reactions to the words protects you. You do not fall into the narcissist's trap, and you do not let the narcissist regain control over your emotions, and in return, the narcissist will slowly lose interest.

The Grey Rock Method

Similar to disengaging emotionally, the grey rock method involves minimizing emotional reactions, but in this case, it is ignoring all interactions, both good and bad. You are aiming to avoid as much interaction as possible, and when you are forced to interact, you should keep it boring and meaningless. The name alludes to a grey rock on the side of the road. Consider how often you notice and remember all of the rocks you walk past in a given day—the answer is most likely none. People do not pay attention to something as mundane and worthless as a grey rock on the side of the road. Your goal in this method is to be as mundane and useless to the narcissist as the grey rock. If you can achieve this state of mediocrity, the narcissist will slowly lose interest in you.

The trick in interacting is to tell you to be robotic in responses. No matter how angry you may feel in response to whatever was said, respond in as few words as possible, and make sure it is never immediately after the message was sent if it does not warrant an immediate response. For example, imagine that he messaged you saying that you are beautiful and he loves you. This should be ignored. Five minutes later, he messages asking how your shared child is doing. Give him the bare minimum answer while still being comprehensive. List what she is doing, whether she is sick, and maybe what she ate for dinner, but keep the interaction as emotionless as possible. Do not emote, no matter how tempting it may be.

Be Realistic

Keeping your interactions with the narcissist realistic will keep you from setting up high standards that she will never meet. Telling yourself that she will never be emotionally supportive with you and that it is a personality limit that she lacks empathy will help you keep reality in mind when dealing with a narcissist. If you are fully prepared for the narcissist to respond in typical narcissist fashion, you will always be prepared, no matter how she responds, and you may even find that you are surprised on occasion. This is key when you are maintaining a relationship with a narcissist, whether romantic, platonic, workplace, familial, or co-parenting. You are protected from the disappointment of narcissistic behavior.

Keep in mind that being realistic does not excuse abuse. It is never okay for someone to hurt you or step on your boundaries. However, if you know that narcissists do those, you will not be as blindsided when it does happen, and you can better prepare in advance to protect yourself. You should absolutely still correct negative or unproductive behaviors, even if it is unpleasant or you would rather avoid doing so.

Focus on the Positive

Likewise, when continuing to interact with a narcissist, remembering to focus on the positive can aid you in recognizing things that you enjoy about the person. After all, something must have attracted you to the narcissist at some point, and you may be happy to see tiny semblances of that person in the narcissist in front of you. While the personality is still likely vastly different from the one you met at first, there still may be parts of the narcissist that at least make her tolerable. For example, she may be horrible at being emotional support or anything but the center of attention, but she may also genuinely be a good cook, and she loves to cook for all of your friends' get-togethers, or she may be incredibly smart and you enjoy the intellectual conversations you have over coffee, even if they involve occasional snide comments about how you do not understand because you did not go to school for politics, or whatever the two of you were discussing. Reminding yourself of the positives can help you in moments when you are ready to lose your temper with the narcissist but it would be detrimental to do so.

Decide Your Hill Die On

The last important tactic to remember is to choose your hill to die on wisely. This is a fancy way of saying choose your battles carefully. Though narcissists seek out confrontation-avoidant people on purpose, choosing to avoid conflict can actually be a way to avoid detection too. For this reason, you should always pick your battles wisely and only be prepared to engage in a conflict if you truly want to deal with the aftermath. While some things are absolutely worthy of a conflict, such as a co-parent choosing to drive with children in the car while drunk, an argument over who said something first is petty, and the narcissist are not likely to ever concede or admit that he is lying. For this reason, you should only choose battles if you are willing to fight for them. If you are unwilling to deal with the aftermath and ultimately, whatever the narcissist did is insignificant, do not bother fighting over it.

Chapter 6

_____ ✦✦✦✦ _____

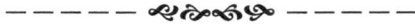

How Did I Get This Way?

Codependency is a part of the reality of an unhealthy bond or relationship that can manifest in a variety of ways, not only in the narcissistic relationship, and will always show up with a narcissistic partner. So, what is codependency anyway, and who is to blame for it?

No one is to blame, and accusing one partner of being more at fault than the other, is just a product of unhealthy relationship dynamics, both with the self and others. By definition, codependency is essentially a condition of behaviors in a relationship in which one partner will facilitate or enable the other partner's irresponsibility, addictive tendencies, mental health issues, immaturity, and even their under-achievement.

Typically, if you are in a codependent partnership with someone, you are likely in need of something from it as well. Oftentimes, the narcissist will need all of the affirmation, accolades, and praise, while the partner is need of someone to take care of and nurture, allowing them to have a sense of fulfillment by meeting someone else's needs.

This can be just as problematic as being a narcissist because it requires that you are dependent upon another person to make you feel worthy of existence. The codependent partnership is just a loop of the same behaviors and patterns being repeated over and over again until someone breaks the pattern. A codependent partner works well with a narcissist because they exist to feel helpful to someone to feel loved for their efforts, and all the narcissist wants is someone to fulfill all of their needs without having to give anything in return.

So, if you are a codependent partner, you may be interested in asking what kinds of traits you might exhibit if you are in that type of personality spectrum.

Characteristics of Codependency

To understand the relationship dynamics prevalent in the narcissistic relationship, having a grasp of the other partner, who is not the narcissist, will be helpful. In the end, it takes two to tango, and if you are in a long-term or even short-term partnership with a narcissist, you might need to start asking the questions of why you might be drawn to that person in the first place.

So, a codependent person will often work to meet the needs of others in the sacrifice of their needs. This act is an assumption of responsibility that is not required but will offer the codependent a sense of purpose, as well as the narcissist someone to meet their every need.

An increase in self-esteem for the codependent comes from controlling their emotions, and by proxy, those of their partner, effectually keeping the peace and making sure that everyone feels satisfied; however, the state of control over emotions prevents the real feelings, issues, or personality disorders from being identified, leading to the behavior loop between the codependent and the narcissist.

Codependents will often feel anxious, worried, or have boundary confusion revolving around intimacy with their partner. This is realized in their attempts to have their needs met by their narcissistic partner who only offers intimacy when it will benefit them, and so the codependent will often have a distorted view of their attractiveness, desire, or right to feel intimacy with their significant other.

One of the greatest indicators of someone being a codependent partner is enmeshment. When you are unable to have authority or autonomy within your relationship, you may decide that you are not whole without the other person and will enmesh yourself in their reality, feelings, and circumstances, blending your realities.

Additionally, codependents will usually, unconsciously, choose partners with addictions, abusive tendencies, mental or emotional disorders or issues, and impulse disorders. These are not the only circumstances, of course, but they are common attributes of a codependent partnership. The reason is that there is a lack of definition of the self, for both the narcissist and the codependent. The codependent feels a sense of self when they are caregiving or controlling another person.

A codependent person will deny their feelings, or that there is anything amiss in the relationship, because of their patterns of thought or belief about what a good partner does for the other. A narcissist will easily convince a codependent that they need to continue to be self-sacrificing, and so, the two work well together to continue manipulating these realities.

Here is a list of some of the common characteristics of a codependent partner and if you or someone you know can check off three or more of these, then you are likely in a codependent state in your partnership:

- Depression

- Compulsive activities (i.e., food binges, shopping sprees, constant house cleaning).

- Holding in emotions

- Constricting feelings

- Anxiety

- In a regular or excessive state of denial

- Overly diligent, of hypervigilant

- Abuse of substances

- Sickness or illness caused by stress or anxiety

- Victim of physical, sexual, or emotional abuse (recurring)

- In a relationship with a person for over two years who has an addiction, without ever asking for help, or seeking therapy

- Can't handle being alone and will make extreme efforts to avoid being alone

- Perfectionism

- Extreme desire for affection and/or acceptance

- Low self-esteem or self-worth

- Feeling a lack of trust

- Dishonesty and/or manipulation

- Overly controlling behavior

- Severe feelings of emptiness and/or boredom

- Intense relationships that are often unstable

- Subordinating your needs for the acceptance of the person you are with

These are some of the hallmarks of a codependent partner, and there are certainly a few more characteristics that can manifest, but these are the core characteristics. You may need to sit down and make a list of some of these qualities and try to determine if these concepts are reflected in your relationship. If so, you will need to understand how a codependent partnership is an unhealthy way to experience love and that there will need to be some shifts and changes in your reality to help you identify your true feelings and desires with your relationship.

Relationship Dynamics of Codependency

A codependent person will often seek out or involve themselves in relationships in which they play a particular role, and it is one that they are the most comfortable with. Their main role is to act as the supportive confidante or rescuer of the other person, and a codependent partner is characterized as being a "helper" type. The reality is that a codependent is dependent on the low, poor, or disordered functioning of their partner to satisfy their emotional sensitivities and needs.

This kind of relationship, especially between a codependent and a narcissist, is colored by lack of healthy boundaries, ineffectual and dysfunctional communication skills, issues with intimacy, patterns of denial, controlling behavior that manifests as caretaking (or various other forms of control), high levels of reactionary behavior, and dependency on these positions.

There is a distinct imbalance in the partnership so that one person is in control, abusive (emotionally/physically/mentally), or enabling, such as in someone else's addiction, immaturity, or in the case of this book, narcissistic tendencies.

The dynamic for a codependent and a narcissist is that one's sense of purpose is to make regular, extreme sacrifices to uphold, or satisfy their partner's needs, while the other maintains the attitude of being superior and worthy of being fawned on and "served" by their partner. Usually, as a result of this dynamic, one partner will lack personal autonomy and self-sufficiency, or authority, while the other will have an overabundance of these qualities to the point of hubris. Some other dynamics include:

- Excessive clinginess

- Needy behaviors

- Dependence on personal fulfillment from their partner

- Mood swings determined by how they perceive their partner currently feels about them (the codependent)

- Self-inflicted self-sacrifice (codependent)

- Getting their partner to "buy into" their vision of life (the narcissist)

- Obedience and attentiveness (the codependent)

- The need to make someone feel important to receive their love in return (the codependent)

- The need to receive love without giving anything in return (the narcissist)

There are a lot of versions of this reality because every relationship is unique and has a beginning, middle, and somewhere, an end. When we are involved with another person, whether or not there is codependency or narcissism, it can be a challenge to maintain your sense of self and reflect through your needs and emotions what you want to support in your relationship.

The codependent and the narcissist share a similar desire or need, but it is reflected in different behaviors. Either way, these dynamics result in unhealthy, imbalanced partnerships that can have a detrimental impact on the core reality of a person's true needs, emotions, and desires. Some people who end up in codependent partnership with a narcissist are empaths, without understanding or knowing this about themselves.

Chapter 7

------ ❦❧ ------

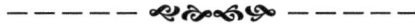

Unlearning Unhealthy Patterns

After going through torture and trauma for many days, narcissistic abuse victims may suffer PTSD commonly referred to as Post Narcissistic Stress Disorder PNSD in this case. Although many individuals may suffer post narcissistic abuse stress disorder, only a few can tell what they are going through. Most victims of narcissistic abuse can barely tell that they have been abused. When they experience stress and anxiety, they relate it to other circumstances in life.

Every individual that has experienced narcissistic abuse at any level must be helped to heal. The people around a person that has experienced abuse must take care of the victim to ensure that he/she gets complete help. Given that most people do not even know that they are suffering, friends and family must help the victims come to terms with reality. Some of the actions done by post abuse victims are subconsciously instigated by their previous experiences. Here are some signs to look out for when dealing with narcissistic abuse victims. These signs are a clear indication that the victim is suffering from PNSD.

- Physical and Emotional Responses to Traumatic Recaps

Victims usually have a way of responding to flashbacks of the traumatic events. In some cases, individuals may undergo deep emotional traumas. A victim suffering from PNSD may start crying for no reason. Remembering the traumatic events they went through may bring back emotions leading to tears, fear, anger disgust, etc. They may also show physical signs of traumatic recap such as shaking and shivering even when they have not been hurt.

- Disturbing Thoughts or Memories

Victims usually experience disturbing memories. A person that has undergone the ordeal of narcissistic abuse may never have peace in life. The stress disorder manifests through disturbing nightmares or visions. The person may start talking in dreams, screaming or wake up sweating. Victims may also hallucinate during the day and keep on seeing images of people trying to hurt them

- Difficulty in Focusing or Falling Sleep

Individuals suffering from post-traumatic stress disorder develop problems with concentration. A victim of narcissistic abuse may find problems focusing on anything for long. They are often found wandering off in their mind. They cannot pay attention at work or school. They are often seen to be in their own world. The patients may stay for long hour's overnight thinking about the trauma. In some cases, insomnia is brought about by the fear of experiencing nightmares related to the ordeal.

- Conflicting Feelings

People who suffer from PTSD are unable to trust themselves or others. They tend to have conflicting feelings due to fear of being hurt again. A PTSD patient may appear to be so much in love in the morning just to start showing remorse and hate a few hours later. If a PTSD patient does not stay with an understanding partner, it often leads to relationship problems. The best medicine for such individuals is reassurance. A person suffering from narcissistic abuse stress must constantly be reassured that the trauma is over and that they're now in safe hands. Given that it takes so many years to publish negativity in the minds of the victims, it also takes a lot of time to wash away the effects. Constant support from family, friends, and colleagues is the best way to get healing for PTSD patients.

- Distorted Sense of Blame

Narcissists train their victims to always find blame for anything happening. As a person stays with a narcissist, he/she becomes the center of blame. The victim is often blamed for failure and success. The victim is never sure what is wrong or right. Every action may lead to abuse even if the victim did the action with good intentions. As the victims try to heal from such trauma, they may show some tendencies of blaming individuals. PTSD patients are quick to blame others to avoid consequences related to the mistake. They are quick to shift blame because they believe the person to blame is the person to be punished. They do all these subconsciously, without thinking about it.

- Social Retreat and Isolation

It is common to see individuals who suffer from stress and anxiety sitting in isolation. Post narcissistic abuse victims also go through the same scenario. In most cases, the victims believe that staying away from people is safer. In other instances, retreat and isolation is a strategy of escaping the shame. As mentioned early, narcissistic abuse patients always blame themselves for the abuse. The patients may find it difficult to associate with people due to the fear of being ridiculed.

- Detach From Reality

Most victims of narcissistic abuse show signs of PTSD by detaching from reality. They avoid tendencies associated with feelings, situations or people. They want to live in a world of their own, where they cannot love or hate. This is a sign of stress disorder associated with traumatic events. The mind subconsciously tries to lock away feelings, tricking the victim to think that lack of feelings is equal to safety. The victim believes that if they do not experience love, they may never have to experience the pain of heartbreak. The victim locks all the feelings that try coming up in order to reduce direct interaction with people. The victim subconsciously assumes that all people are evil and associating with them may eventually result in painful experiences.

- Hyper-Vigilance

Individuals suffering from PNSD show fear and anxiety. They are easily startled and angered. They may be angered by the smallest of actions. They may also be frightened if someone appears from behind or by hearing a loud sound. Most of the victims are always on the lookout; they are in a desperate need to have a 360-degree view of their environment. When thy are in the house, they prefer locking all doors and windows. They may be frightened even at the sound of movement made by an insect. They always look at strangers critically and may respond aggressively to people they do not know. All these factors are indications of stress and anxiety that is deeply rooted in the trauma experienced during narcissistic abuse.

- Fear or Panic for No Apparent Reasons

Individuals suffering from traumatic stress disorder often show fear. They may show fear even when there is nothing threatening around. They are usually afraid of the unknown and often panic when in stress or left alone. They are very protective of everything they find valuable such as children. They are always afraid that everyone around has intentions to harm or to steal anything they own.

- Inconsistent or Conflicting Beliefs

Most post narcissistic abuse victims are never sure of what is true and what is false. They do not have firm ideologies to believe in. They constantly waiver their thoughts and end up believing what people say. Most patients tend to lack self-esteem since that have been made to believe they are not worthy. Even when they try coming to terms with the fact that they are just victims, the idea does not stay around for long. Most victims easily find themselves going back to old thoughts.

How to Analyze People

Everyone can be a victim of narcissistic abuse. The first line of defense for all victims is having the ability to analyze people. By analyzing individuals, a person is in a position to tell whether someone is narcissistic or not.

Parents

In the case of parents, the victims are more often unfortunate. Being born or adopted by a narcissistic parent is the most unfortunate thing that could happen to anyone. In this case, the victims are unable to analyze people or to make any decision. They are innocent and vulnerable. In the case of parents, it is the neighbors or other family members that may be able to spot narcissism and rescue the child. However, as a person matures, he/she might be able to spot narcissistic tendencies in parents. Narcissistic parents are abusive and controlling even when their children are adults. They control a person's life to the extent of choosing a life partner. If you feel that your parent has some narcissistic tendencies, analyze their motives in every action. Narcissistic parents use their children to achieve pride. They punish their children for failure and demand that the children maintain high standards that the narcissist deems success.

Partner

Since most narcissistic abuse victims are romantic partners, it is important for all people to have a third eye when dating. Some clues can help a person spot narcissism in their partner. First, narcissists idealize their partner. If you happen to date someone that is 100% ideal for you in all ways, be careful.

Another very clear sign of narcissism is obsession and possessiveness. Narcissistic individuals do not give up on pursuing a person. They do not take no for an answer and keep on coming with enticing gifts. They may show desperation and even manipulate the victim just to have them.

The next sign of narcissism in relationships is separation. The narcissist separates the victim from friends and family. If you are in a relationship and realize that you are being separated from friends and family, start being critical.

Spot this pattern and stay vigilant every time you start a new relationship. It starts with Idealization then obsession, separation, and abuse. These are the most common and visible factors to observe to avoid getting trapped in narcissistic relationships.

Friends

In friendship, narcissists only come in for social or material gain. If you suspect that you are in a narcissistic friendship, ask yourself what could it be that the person wants from you. Narcissists often fail to hide their true intentions. If you look closely, you may be able to realize that a person only associates with you because of your wealth or status. Such individuals may sound genuine at first, but manipulation soon crops in. To avoid falling into such traps, cut links to such individuals.

Avoid creating long-lasting bonds or making investments together with an individual you do not know well.

Children

Children can be narcissistic too. As a parent, you have to analyze your child for tendencies of narcissism. Unfortunately, most parents groom narcissism in children. Narcissistic children may come out as confident, assertive, and natural leaders. The parent has to help the child realize that they are not better than the rest of the world. On the contrary, most parents encourage their children by telling them that they are the best. If narcissism can be spotted in a child at an early age, the parents may be able to help the child. It is easy to help a child learn their true personality and get rid of any fears. In many instances, narcissists are just afraid of the unknown and have low self-esteem. Being able to help someone understand that failure is part of life and being weak is okay helps the person start accepting their true personality. They eventually get rid of the self-glorified false personality and live their life according to the truth.

How to Deal With a Narcissistic Partner

Dealing with a narcissistic partner is not a walk in the park. The best way is to spot the signs and avoid falling into the trap. However, if you realize that you are already in the trap, you need to be very technical in your escape strategy. Running from the hands of a narcissist is never easy. The abuser will keep on pursuing you and using manipulation to have you on their side. To deal with a narcissistic partner, follow this basic guide:

Basic Guide to Recognize and Handle Narcissists

Step 1: Gain Knowledge

The first step to dealing with a narcissist is gaining knowledge. Do extensive research by reading books such as this one and watching videos. Gaining knowledge will help you understand every principle used and applied by narcissists. If you are already in a narcissistic relationship, you must be careful in your quest to gain knowledge. The narcissistic partner should never know you are gaining such knowledge. Make sure you clear your browser history after searching such topics online. If the partner realizes that you are gaining knowledge on the subject, he /she may block all the possible ways of gaining such knowledge.

Step 2: Understand the Cycle

Understanding the narcissistic abuse cycle will help you know where you stand. If you are not in a narcissistic relationship, the knowledge of the cycle will help you avoid falling into the trap. If you are already in a narcissistic relationship, understanding the cycle will help you know the phase of abuse you are at.

Step 3: Learn to Analyze People

It is not possible to escape a narcissist if you do not know how to play the mind games. Narcissists thrive on mind games. You must find a way out by playing the games better than the narcissist. Emotional intelligence is a whole subject on its own. Invest in learning emotional intelligence. Learn to study people's emotions and manage them. Start understanding the actions that narcissists take and what makes them take such actions. Once you understand analyzing people, you will be ready to beat the narcissist at his/her own game.

Step 4: Mend Relationships

Narcissists are often successful because they manage to alienate their victims. If you choose to mend fences with friends and family, you may have someone to trust. After you finally understand that a narcissist only intents to hurt and harm, you must be able to retrace your route. Find people you can trust and those who trust your words. Find the people who love you genuinely. If you have not yet been captured by a narcissist, your first clue is to always maintain friendships. No matter how sweet the relationship may sound, make sure you maintain friendships and family relationships. Do not let a new person in your life take over your relationships or control the way you interact with people.

Step 5: With Help from Friends and Family Uncover the Narcissist

The only way to escape the traps of a narcissist forever is to ensure that the truth goes out. You must ensure that there is sufficient evidence to convict the abuser for the crimes committed. You should also ensure that the community and people around believe everything you say about this person. One reason why narcissists never get caught is that they create a very self-righteous public image. In some cases, they are powerful individuals with respected leadership roles in society. When you say your word against theirs, you might not be recognized.

To ensure that your word holds ground, you must first get some incriminating evidence. Gather evidence by the help of friends and family. Look for people who may have your best interests at heart. You may even be required to stay in the abusive relationship a lot longer in your quest to find the right information. Collect written, video and audio evidence. To ensure that the abuse does not notice your actions, you must be skillful and use help from close friends. When you eventually decide to stand up to the abuser, be sure you have evidence to convince the entire community. If you give the abuser a chance to escape they may be very manipulative with their words. Make sure you show their personality publicly so that they do not have anywhere else to hide.

Your Brain in the Abusive Relationship

The brain is the most affected part of your body when you are in an abusive relationship. As already mentioned, the pain threshold for physical and emotional abuses on the brain is the same. This means that any emotional or physical abuse directly affects the brain. The key to surviving any traumatic events and abuses is protecting the brain. Any individual who undergoes narcissistic abuse can only survive by protecting the brain from the trauma. If you are in a relationship that keeps inflicting pain, you must find a way of protecting the brain.

The only way to protect the brain is learning the truth. Emotionally intelligent people know how to differentiate facts from fiction. If you can train your brain to know the truth and live in reality, you will have very strong mental power. In fact, narcissists are not in a position to break anyone who stays within their mind. The first thing anyone in the clear state of mind should understand is that the narcissist is a liar. You must understand that the narcissist thrives on lies and capitalizes on your emotions. The narcissist hurts the emotions to make the victim feel worthless.

If you know what the narcissist is trying to do, you will not allow your brain to accept the message. You must train your brain to reject such negative information and only accept positive information. You must train your brain to only accept what is true and reject what is a lie.

Protecting your brain during narcissistic abuse also depends on your ability to control emotions. If you can differentiate between the truth and lies, you will not be affected by lies. If a narcissist keeps saying you are stupid, you will not be affected by their words because you know clearly, you are wise. The only fighting chance any individual has in a narcissistic relationship is staying sober. This includes the ability to make decisions that are not influenced by emotions.

As a victim, you must know that you are being victimized. You should be able to analyze your abuser and understand that he/she is suffering from a mental disorder. You should be in a position to analyze the personality disorder and start capitalizing on the abuser's weaknesses. You should be in a position to unravel the hidden personality of the abuser and shame their ego.

Although maintaining mental stability in such situations is not easy, every person can control their minds. If you have something you stand for, start from that point. Although narcissists distort a person's way of thinking, there are a few constants that remain. Every victim must be able to recognize the available constants and start utilizing them to overcome mental trauma. For instance, a narcissist may sabotage a person's path to success but they may never sabotage a person's past achievements. Even if he/she makes you believe you are incompetent, find one thing you can do very well.

Start building your strength and confidence from that aspect. Start reaffirming your thoughts and abilities. You must be in a position to remember your past success before you met your abuser. Think of the important steps you made in life and the milestones you have achieved. Remembering your old self gives you the desire to want to achieve again.

The victim must also be on a constant quest to enrich their brains. Feed your brain with the right information. The victim must ensure that the positive ideas that go into the mind outweigh the negative ideas that the abuser tries to instill. The victim should enjoy reading books, watching TV, playing mental stimulation games and d keeping up with the trends. Gaining knowledge that the abuser lacks puts the victim in a position of control. The victim can counteract negative energy being built by the abuser.

The victim starts differentiating facts from lies. The abuser may try to sabotage every effort made to gain knowledge. However, we live in an era of freedom. Every person has the freedom to gain knowledge. Even if you are confined to a house, you can still gain knowledge by reading books and magazines.

Chapter 8

------- ❧❦❧ -------

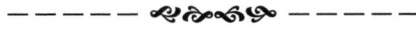

Can I Choose a New Way of Thinking?

Life may not be all sunshine and roses for victims who manage to escape narcissistic abuse cycles. Many struggle to heal for years afterward, experiencing intermittent periods of growth and rehabilitation peppered with bouts of emotional relapse. Even so, recovering victims often report an overwhelming feeling of relief and a surreal sense of calm once they start to get used to the rhythm of their lives under the rules of No-Contact with dangerous narcissists.

Even through the difficult periods, it's important for any victim to consistently forgive themselves, appreciate their own strength and resilience, and throw themselves enthusiastically into a self-care routine. They must also try to consistently look towards the future rather than ruminating too heavily on the painful past. The most insidious legacy of narcissistic abuse is that it attempts to corrupt the victim's ability to enjoy self-esteem, interpersonal love, and all the other beautiful things that an empathetic life can offer, even after the abusive situation has been left behind. The best and most powerful form of revenge you can seek upon a narcissistic abuser is to deny them that possibility. Take the reins of your life; make the conscious choice to be happy and compassionate; give and receive honest, authentic love with joy and optimism. Don't allow your victimhood to define you.

Hypersensitivity

Many victims of narcissists are already self-identified empaths, or highly sensitive people (HSPs) before they even meet the narcissist in question. Some, though, only become awakened to this reality after leaving the narcissistic relationship or regime.

Hypersensitivity comes in many forms and varying degrees of intensity. Many people grow to see it as a superpower, though it needs consistent training, rest and care, just like a muscle. Intensive boundary work is a necessity for empaths, as is the establishment and maintenance of a self-care routine. It does not need to be costly--it simply needs to remind the victim on a regular basis that they are worthy of care and attention, and that they are responsible for creating their own happiness.

Some unfortunate victims may not find the support that they need in healing from this abuse. Many empaths and HSPs find themselves in frequent conflict with highly individualistic people, who invalidate their experiences of narcissistic abuse by calling them normal, and dismissing their feelings as overreactions. They might advise the victim to "grow a thicker skin" or to "toughen up," whether or not they realize that these words essentially serve to blame the victim for the abuse inflicted upon them.

If this happens to you, remind yourself of the person you were before the abuse started. You were not perfect--no one is--but you were strong. You were your own person. There was nothing wrong with you. You didn't deserve to be targeted, manipulated, exploited, shamed, or used as an emotional punching bag.

Try to remind yourself that the person who's telling you to toughen up may mean well, but that they are ignorant. They might buy into the "just world" fallacy--the idea that people get what they deserve in life, so people who are suffering have usually done something to deserve this punishment--and lack the perspective necessary to provide you with helpful advice. While this can be extremely frustrating, or infuriating if it's happening repeatedly, try not to bear anger towards these people. Put yourself in their shoes.

Imagine two empty water glasses set down on a table top with standard force; one stays unaffected by the impact, while the other shatters. It would be easy to deduce that there was something inherently defective in the glass that broke. But what if you came to learn that the intact glass had previously been cocooned in bubble wrap, while the broken glass had been repeatedly heated and cooled and then struck with a mallet, forming thousands of tiny invisible cracks?

A victim of prolonged narcissistic abuse is a shell of a person, a glass with thousands of tiny invisible cracks throughout. They need to be handled gently for a while, in order to heal. They may not be able to handle adversity that most people can take in stride. But that doesn't mean they started out defective; it means they are in need of repair, and patient understanding.

One place where this analogy fails, though, is in the aftermath; unlike a broken glass, a hypersensitive victim can mend all those little cracks, and eventually come out even stronger than the glass that was protected by bubble wrap all along. Empaths and HSPs can grow into emotional warriors, beacons for other victims in need of role models, and powerful healers. Hypersensitivity does not make people weak; it teaches them incredible strength.

Imagine those two glasses side by side again. This time, you're fully aware of what each has been through, and the abused glass does not break. Now, which one do you find more impressive?

Echoism

Echoism is defined as a phobia of narcissistic traits within the self. It's common in victims of severe narcissistic abuse, who become afraid of expressing their own needs, appearing selfish, or receiving special attention of any kind, most often because the narcissist in their life would punish them for doing these things.

One important test for victims of narcissistic abuse is this: are you able to enjoy your own company for a day, or a full weekend perhaps, without having an emotional meltdown? If not, there's no need to feel ashamed, but it may be wise to seek help for further recovery. There's nothing at all wrong with being social, but victims of narcissistic abuse may use their busy social and professional lives to distract themselves from unresolved pain or difficult emotional sensations that need to be addressed. Victims also are typically trained to be codependent, which means they may struggle to make decisions, grasp their true opinions and preferences, or even recognize their own emotions, without a dominant personality present to dictate these things for them.

Isolation can be painful and challenging, but it can also be a powerful tool for emotional growth or spiritual awakening. When you choose it for yourself, rather than having it thrust upon you, it can be extraordinarily empowering.

Stay mindful of the fact that this is your life, no one else's, and it's entirely possible that you only get one of those to live through. Make sure you're living it for yourself--not to please some ungrateful and apathetic narcissist.

Reframing memories

Unfortunately, victims of narcissistic abuse are often haunted by an unfounded sense of shame, even after they've cut ties and moved on from the narcissist who hurt them. It's important to work with someone--a therapist, counselor, healer, or spiritual guide--to reframe your memories of the relationship you shared with the narcissist, to start to untangle and alleviate the stress of this shame.

One especially effective technique that narcissistic abusers use is to react to a victim's bid for equal and fair treatment as though it is an unreasonable and narcissistic request. The narcissist's voice may haunt the victim, even long after they've cut ties, asking: "Just who do you think you are?" or "It's always about you, isn't it?" This is a combination of projection and gaslighting that can truly disrupt the victim's ability to assert or defend themselves in life. They become paralyzed with self-conscious fear, struggle to advocate for their own personal interests, and often get stuck in a cycle of further generosity towards the narcissist, all in a vain attempt to prove their own capacity for empathy. Somehow, by trying to stand up for themselves, the victims are tricked into bowing down yet again, and even more deeply, to the narcissist.

So when the relationship is over, the victim is left carrying the shame of the abusive behavior that they tolerated, as well as the shameful fear that they were somehow guilty of the same narcissistic behavior that their abuser displayed. This can impact the victim's future relationships, smothering confidence and promoting phantom anxiety.

If feelings of shame are haunting you, the best thing you can do for yourself is find a therapist or counselor to help you reframe your memories and rewrite your narrative. You'll need an objective third party to help you see the parts of your own memories that you've gotten into the habit of blinding yourself to: namely, the parts where your abuser crossed lines, and treated you in dehumanizing ways. These memories can be extremely painful, which is why many victims' brains automatically edit them out, or alter them, for the sake of self-protection. Victims should not expect to be exclusively self-reliant during their recovery processes; a good support system full of empathetic people with good judgment and strong moral character will be necessary, and the assistance of a licensed mental health professional should be included if it is at all possible.

Reconnecting with Your True Self

In the long term, purging narcissism from your life feels a bit like taking off a corset that you've been wearing your whole life and never even knew it. On the one hand, there's an enormous sense of relief, and the sudden ability to breathe more deeply than you ever realized you could. On the other hand, this corset may have been holding in some unsightly baggage that now is free to roll around and bounce and jiggle. This corset also may have been masking some pain that you've been normalizing for years, pain which now suddenly feels unbearable. And everything mundane that you never used to think about, like how to hold your rib cage when you walk, stand, or sit? Now, you find you have to think long and hard about every move you make, because everything feels so unfamiliar, foreign and awkward.

Removing narcissism from your life frees you from a lot of toxic nonsense, but it also sometimes means getting rid of your emotional safety net, which can be very scary. Without these dominant personalities around to tell you what to do, how to think, and how to feel, you'll have to decide for yourself, and take responsibility for your own behaviors. Reconnecting with your authentic self--the person you were before the abuse rewired your brain--can be a lengthy process, so you might as well dive in and do your best to enjoy it. Ask yourself: what do

I like, when no one else is telling me what I'm supposed to live? What do I detest? Where do I want to be? How do I want to feel? How do I want to designate my time?

The most important question to ask yourself is what you want. Guided meditation practice can be enormously helpful in pondering that question, as well as silencing all the voices in your head that aren't your own. Society is full of narcissistic talking heads, telling us all what we are supposed to want, and what goals are worth striving for. But if you ignore them, you can open yourself up to a world of possibilities. For example, what if you really don't want to be wealthy? What if all you want is to be happy, healthy, and financially comfortable enough to give back to charities, or to friends in need? What if you don't actually want to dominate your career field, or maintain an athlete's body, or gain a million followers in social media? What if you haven't found your joy yet, simply because you were led to search for it in all the wrong places?

Encourage yourself to experiment; try new things, and be bold. You may be quite surprised at the person you find underneath all those emotional bruises and baggage once they've been cleared away.

Healing and Moving Forward

Forgiveness is an important part of your healing process. But you do not necessarily want to forgive your abuser. In fact, many victims of narcissistic abuse are too forgiving of narcissists, which is why they allowed the abuse to last as long as it did.

The person you need to forgive is yourself. First, acknowledge that the truth of your story has been obscured in your head for a long time; the narcissist was not a good person, and did not have your best interests at heart. It was all an act. They knew you were in pain, and instead of releasing you from it, they compounded it at every possible opportunity. You played into this because you wanted to see the best in them. You trusted and believed in them. You did nothing wrong to deserve this treatment. You deserve forgiveness.

But at the same time, on some level, you had to be aware that this relationship was unhealthy, and you allowed it to continue anyway. You put up with behaviors that you should have walked away from. You made excuses for your abuser and protected them from facing the consequences of their actions. This is where you begin to take personal responsibility for your healing, which is not to be confused with accepting blame for the abuse. Your goal here is not to make yourself feel bad, or convince yourself that you asked for this treatment; on the contrary, your goal is to try and understand why you allowed the abuse to happen, so that you can make better, healthier choices moving forward. There is no shame in this; usually, we accept abusive behaviors because they come alongside other things that we desperately desire, such as a sense of security, financial empowerment, or simply a feeling of significance. Many of us long to feel needed by someone, and it's that simple desire that leaves us vulnerable to narcissistic abuse. Recognizing your own points of vulnerability--the ones that continuously encouraged you to ignore the red flags and remain in a toxic relationship--is the best way to guard yourself against future threats of abuse.

Finally, you may feel stuck, paralyzed, or pulled in two different directions for quite some time after leaving a narcissistic abuser. Half of your soul will be drifting into the gravitational pull of the past, wanting to revisit memories and explore them, looking for answers. Meanwhile, the other half will be exhausted of this situation and eager to move forward, leaving the abuse behind like a snake shedding its skin. Understand that this dichotomy will tire you out quickly, so it may be best to set up designated timeframes to explore the past (therapy, meditation, or even just planned chats with trusted friends) and the future separately, allowing you to devote your full attention to each and live mindfully in the present.

Eventually, you will reach a point where you are able to meet new people, and you won't feel the need to explain what you've been through in order to justify your personality or behaviors. You may not be conscious of it, or see it happening, but when you get there, you will have officially freed yourself from the claws of narcissistic abuse. Don't forget your story, but recognize this as an opportunity to write a new ending, and change the entire narrative. And always remember that the abuse you've suffered through never made you weak--it only served to make you stronger, smarter, and more powerful in the end.

Chapter 9

————— ✂❧❧☙❧ —————

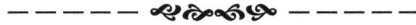

Does Genetics Play a Role?

This section first reviews the common phases of a narcissistic relationship – idealize, devalue and discard – touches on the common traits of victims and reasons individuals enter, willingly or unwillingly, into narcissistic relationships. Note: it's just as important to understand what drives people to these relationships as it is to understand what they've grown unwilling to accept.

Often, victims are so manipulated and accustomed to the abusive circumstances that recovery never comes. They experience years of abuse without fully realizing the severity of their situation. In the most severe cases, the victims believe, without question, that they're actually the problem and grow dependent on the possibility of their captor providing genuine and needed intimacy and bonding that never occurs. They're left confused and feeling powerless, constantly attempting to change their circumstances and left sorely disappointed.

Finally, this section culminates with tips to leave a narcissist, what to expect when one decides to move on, and ways to rebuild and renew.

Narcissists and Relationships - The Victim's False Life

Living with someone that suffers from Narcissistic Personality Disorder is extremely confusing, disheartening, painful and downright debilitating. Victims are propelled to extreme highs, and equally extreme lows caught on a never-ending roller coaster of emotions without the means of getting off safely. They may feel as if they're stuck in a revolving doorway with no clear way to exit.

Sufferers go through a very specific set of relational stages, which, although more common than most expect, are actually very difficult for the victims themselves to recognize objectively and then manage to escape. These individuals are often caught completely off guard when the narcissist's mask comes off, having believed they were relating to someone who is immensely charming, charismatic and by all outward appearances 'perfect'.

Once the mask is removed, however, trust dissolves and the victims are affected deeply. They must learn to adjust their entire thought process, rethinking everything they knew to be true. Their lives are turned completely upside down and they are left reaching for nonexistent safety, a net no longer there, or that never really existed. There's a period of time, often prolonged, in which the victim feels lost—paralyzed as if they can no longer trust themselves or their judgment. And, since true narcissists are unable to feel empathy, it's only their victims who suffer once the red flags go up, leaving these individuals feeling even more lonely and desperate.

The narcissist is unable to believe that they've caused pain, and can't relate emotionally to their victim. They'll suggest their victim is crazy, thereby relieving themselves of any potential guilt. Extreme narcissists are typically unable to feel healthy emotions at all towards other people. They believe others, their entire network of family, friends, and acquaintances, are there simply to serve their needs. These people are not human beings; they're objects, there to provide narcissistic supply.

It's this inability to look inward that makes most narcissists unwilling to seek therapy. They're rarely the ones to seek out help with their relationships or initiate professional treatment. The victims are usually the seekers. What's most disheartening is that the victims often seek help for their own perceived mental imbalances, which the narcissist has convinced them they possess. It takes a highly intuitive therapist and one skilled in NPD to identify the true underlying issues, bring to light possible narcissistic abuse, and effectively help the victim cope and rebuild.

If the victim convinces their narcissistic spouse to seek couples counseling, danger to their well-being may actually increase. An untrained counselor could fall victim to the narcissist's charm, leading to further disillusionment and self-esteem issues in the victim. The narcissist learns what triggers their victim to confide in others regarding her unhappiness and 'up their game', ensuring they work twice as hard the next time to keep their victim quiet.

It's difficult for therapists to identify narcissistic abuse and have the victim believe it's happened to them, for the victim to self-identify and for the therapist to secure their trust once their world falls apart. Well qualified therapists and successfully revived victims care are few and far between. A therapist needs to play detective and understand that the reason the victim believes they're seeking treatment may actually be an unhealthy consequence (i.e., anxiety, depression, stress, etc.) of a larger problem.

Therapists must be patient in working with potential abuse victims, not only getting them to accept that they've been abused and working with them on a plan to move forward but ultimately, within this process, helping them to better understand themselves and why they fell victim in the first place. In doing so, the cycle is less likely to repeat itself.

It's ultimately up to the victim to vocalize an understanding of what's occurred and gather the strength to move forward. Eventually, they may be willing to help other sufferers of narcissistic abuse, so that the condition is reduced nearly to the point of elimination. The cycle must be broken, and only those who have witnessed it have the power to help prevent it.

Supply and Demand

The NPD relationship is a constant supply and demand struggle. Think simple economics. The narcissistic supply runs low as the demand for it increases within the narcissist and they need more attention. As the supply depletes, energy depletes in the victim, and the victim is unable to meet the demand. This causes the narcissist to explode. In the aftermath, the supply is refueled as control is reestablished and the victim is re-motivated to provide the needed reserves.

A narcissist shows no remorse for the terrible things they do. They never say sorry, but they'll hang out, still wanting desperately to be needed, or, at the very least, not discarded. If one summons the courage to leave and is successful, the narcissist will continue to insert themselves into the victim's life, hoovering to refuel their supply. They'll piece-meal the return of personal possessions if he still has access to them, and he may continue to do so for years to come, long after they're forgotten. As long as they're demanding attention and the victim is supplying it by allowing contact, this pattern will continue.

Chapter 10

──────── ✥❧✤✤ ────────

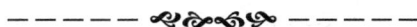

Freedom at Last

In order to understand why you keep attracting toxic people in your life, you have to understand why you keep allowing that kind of treatment. Typically, this starts in childhood. Maybe you had a narcissistic mother who, no matter what you did, was simply never satisfied. Therefore, you developed a people-pleasing persona in order to fulfill what was lacking. There are two traits that are necessary in a person that manipulators look for—someone with a conscience as well as someone who has excessive deference.

People who have a conscience are less likely to hurt others, meaning that a narcissist will feel comfortable manipulating them since they will technically allow it to happen. If someone believes in love, they are less likely to remove themselves from a toxic situation since they may have been taught not to do that or that they can get through anything. In the same sense, someone who is a people pleaser will agree to a lot of what the narcissist wants or needs since they want to make them happy.

On one hand, there is a narcissist that looks for people who are vulnerable to be taken advantage of, and on the other hand, there are people who are wounded and try to please everyone to make themselves happy. Both make a very toxic situation.

So, how can this be avoided? In a sense, it is difficult to predict as it depends mostly on how educated people are about narcissists and empaths. If we see that someone's spouse is toxic and abusive, we may open up to them and tell them. The typical response may be a bunch of excuses to dismiss the behavior, or maybe the victim has already researched the behaviors but is still hopeful that their partner may change. Hope is the word that keeps many in situations where they do not belong.

In order to correct or stop yourself from being manipulated, you first have to understand how people might manipulate you. There are seven ways people manipulate, and they include:

1. They place blame,

2. They make you feel insecure,

3. They use self-pity,

4. They flatter you,

5. They subtly intimidate you,

6. They create a false discord, and

7. They play dumb.

They place blame. This type is generally a silent form of manipulation. If someone is blamed over and over again, they will then take on that burden and apologize for everything. If your behavior is being judged, that is also another form of manipulation since they are trying to make you feel bad about who you are. If someone is telling you whether what you are doing is good or bad, that is a telltale sign of abuse.

They make you feel insecure. If you are insecure, then you can be easily manipulated since they will belittle you any chance they get. In this instance, they will also criticize you, which could leave you second-guessing your every move. They may also try to confuse you by turning little mistakes into really big mistakes.

They use self-pity. There are people on this planet that will pity themselves and will have sob stories about how terrible their life is. This is to get you hooked into helping them, and if they know you are a kind and caring person, they will try to manipulate that by using their pity parties.

They will flatter you. Flattery cannot always be believed since it could be used to get you to lower your guard to make you susceptible to manipulation. When someone does flatter you, they will earn your goodwill; however, this is not always with good intentions in mind. If you know yourself well, you will be more likely to combat this type of manipulation as you will be able to tell when someone is being fake.

They will subtly intimidate you. This is done in a subtle way, such as telling you that a certain behavior is dangerous. They will tell you that you should act a certain way in different situations. This is to imply that if you do not act a certain way, you will end up with a less-than-desirable outcome. This manipulation tactic is used to instill fear in you.

They create a false discord. If someone is always up in arms over little things, you are most likely being manipulated. This will keep you on edge, and you will wonder what you are doing wrong at any given moment. Manipulators do this to try to condition people to treat them a certain way or they will act out. This manipulation tactic is typically used to avoid any accountability, consequence, or punishment.

They will play dumb. People will play dumb to get out of doing work because someone else does it better. For instance, if a husband does not want to load the dishwasher, he will tell his wife that she is better at it. If someone pretends not to understand you, they are also trying to manipulate you by not taking accountability for an issue they are involved with.

All of these manipulation tactics will lead to toxic and dishonest relationships. If you recognize that someone is trying to manipulate you, it may be best to call them out on it so they may recognize the behavior. Chances are, if they truly are toxic, they will not own up to it anyway, which leaves you to run the other way.

Codependent Or Empath?

Codependent and empath are often used interchangeably; however, they are both different in the ways that they seek out validation, love, and understanding. Empaths can have codependent traits, but not all codependents can be empaths. Codependents are always looking to fix and help people, while empaths are spiritually in tune with how other people are feeling and absorb other people's energy. Both want to be loved, validated, and understood; however, they both react differently to narcissists.

Empath

An empath will typically bolt at any sign of a narcissist. The only way they will feel stuck in a place with a narcissist is if they were too young to understand the red flags or they were not educated on narcissists or empath relationships. When an empath is educated on the subject, or has been hurt by a narcissist and has done their own research, they are more likely to get out of toxic situations. Empaths have some of the following traits:

1. They absorb others' emotions,

2. They are highly sensitive and intuitive,

3. They are able to see a point of view from all angles, and

4. They deeply understand people, places, and things.

Narcissists do not have empathy, so they tend to latch onto empaths in order to feed off of them to fulfill that need. Empaths do have a lot to give; however, they get exhausted and drained very quickly. The good aspect of an empath is that they will recognize what is using their energy and decide to distance themselves from that source. So, if an empath has a narcissistic husband, there will be times when the empath has to pull away and isolate for a while in order to recharge. Empaths are very aware of themselves and their surroundings, and that will give them the upper hand as they will call out the narcissist's behavior.

Codependent

Codependents will waste their entire lives with a narcissist thinking that they can fix them or help them change. There may come a time when a codependent is fed up and wants out, but they are usually held in the relationship because of guilt from giving up on someone. Codependents have the following traits:

1. They have low self-esteem,

2. They look outside of themselves for validation,

3. They are fixers and helpers,

4. They attach to an alpha personality for identity,

5. Their mood is dependent on the mood of the alpha, and

6. They are looking for praise and have a desire to be liked.

A narcissist is not as afraid of a codependent as they are an empath, so codependents are the most sought after for a narcissist. Codependents have a poor sense of boundaries, so they may be easily taken advantage of, and once they try to enforce boundaries, they will notice severe resistance. It is difficult for a codependent to break free from a narcissist because they cannot see themselves separate from them.

The following chart will show the differences side by side, which may be easier to pinpoint exactly which one you might be:

Empath	Codependent
I can sit with your suffering	I want to and can fix you
I am comfortable with a variety of emotions	I have an emotional addiction and feed off people's emotions
I see why you believe, think, and feel the ways that you do	I want to believe, think, and feel the things that you do
I hold a space for your emotions	I want to take on your emotions like they are my own
My relationships are typically fulfilling	I tend to be taken advantage of and constantly feel drained from it

Let's picture the two in relationships. There is a narcissistic husband plus an empath wife and a narcissistic husband and a codependent wife. The empath wife, when she recognizes the signs of abuse, will be aware of her surroundings and will call out the behaviors since she will not put up with feeling drained from it. The codependent wife will recognize the signs but will think the problem is her, which will enable the husband to act as he does. Thus, the codependent will stay in the relationship and will continue to make excuses for why they are staying in a bad situation. An empath can have codependent traits, but unless the empath is drained beyond belief, they will have the strength and knowledge to step away from what is toxic to them.

How A Trauma Bond Is Formed

A trauma bond is formed over time, and it tends to keep victims in the relationships because they are hoping it will get back to the "good" phase. The main goal of an abuser is to continue to receive some sort of benefit from you. When you are completely drained and exhausted, they may become angry that you cannot fulfill the supply that they need at the time. You will then try to work harder to please your abuser and keep the relationship afloat. When someone says "it isn't always bad, there are good times too," they are typically living in this type of cycle in their relationship. There are signs that you have a trauma bond with your abuser, and here are the top five:

1. You constantly feel tired.

2. You feel like you can do nothing right for the narcissist.

3. If you do try to leave, the angst of losing them pulls you back.

4. You know they will cause you more pain, you are waiting for it, yet you allow it to occur.

5. You put them as a priority. If they text you, you will drop everything to reply.

Trauma bonds are typically found in relationships that have an inconsistent reinforcement and they may even be referred to as the Stockholm Syndrome. Stockholm Syndrome is typically seen in prisoners of war or hostage situations. Over time, an abusive relationship will take the shape of Stockholm Syndrome, and the victims will actually protect, love, and depend on their abuser to survive. When the victim has completely disassociated (numbed) themselves from the pain of the situation, they start to feel helpless then fantasize about their abuser.

The type of environment needed to foster a trauma bond has "intensity, complexity, inconsistency, and a promise, [and] victims stay because they are holding on to that elusive 'promise' or hope" (Stines, 2015). When a relationship begins in a way that creates a good feeling or environment, the victim is always waiting for it to get back to that point. This is what will keep someone stagnant in a situation much longer than they should be because they keep hoping it will go back.

There are ways to recover from a toxic trauma bond. The primary six ways to recover include the following:

1. Focus on making decisions that support your self-care,

2. Learn how to grieve,

3. Get used to understanding your emotions,

4. Build healthy connections in your life,

5. Make a list of behaviors that you will not accept, and

6. Live one day at a time.

Focus on making decisions that support your self-care. In other words, do not make any decisions that are going to hurt you. You may be feeling weak from the trauma, and the last thing you should do is talk negatively to yourself or relive what you have just experienced. Be nice to yourself and allow your body and mind the time to process all that has happened.

Learn how to grieve. Losing a marriage or relationship that was different than you thought it initially was will be like losing a loved one. You need to allow yourself time to grieve the loss.

Get used to understanding your emotions. When someone is in a toxic trauma bond, they tend to think in the way they are manipulated into thinking. Thus, it will take time to detox from that mindset and think on your own. Allow yourself time to feel all of the emotions so you are able to process them and own them.

Build healthy connections in your life. The only way to create healthy connections is to eliminate unhealthy connections. Find who you have a strong bond with, without any drama, and invest in those relationships.

Make a list of behaviors that you will not accept. You have accepted immoral behavior for too long. Make a list of behaviors that you vow never to accept again and follow through with it. For example, I will manage my own finances or I will not argue with someone who calls me names.

Live one day at a time. There will be good days and bad days, so make sure to live each day like it is a fresh start. Do not focus on the bad days; focus on moving forward and getting your life back.

In order to detox from a trauma bond, it is important to be away from that person with no contact. It is not until then that the victim will see the devastation that they have endured for so long; once that is seen, the healing process will begin.

Coping-Mechanisms For Narcissistic Abuse

Coping mechanisms can be used either when in an abusive relationship or when coping with the aftermath of the abuse. We will explore coping mechanisms for those that are still in the cycle of abuse to try to help them step out of it. Many of these can also apply to after the relationship has ended as well.

1. Make yourself a priority and focus on improving your physical and mental health,

2. Create and enforce boundaries,

3. Understand that you cannot fix an abusive person,

4. Do not blame yourself,

5. Do not engage with an abusive person, and

6. Work on creating an exit plan.

Make yourself a priority and focus on improving your physical and mental health. Instead of worrying about pleasing your abuser, focus on yourself. It may seem odd at first, or you may feel guilty, but you need to take care of yourself in order to function and stay healthy. Sleep is also very important as your body is most likely stressed all of the time and you need to be able to recover.

Create and enforce boundaries. Even if you did not have boundaries before, you need to create a list of boundaries for the abuser. Then, you need to enforce them. For instance, the abuser goes through your phone without permission. Add a passcode on your phone and let them know that it is not respectful to do that and if they need to see your phone, you can unlock it for them. That is just one example; another would be that they are not to insult you or call you names or else the conversation will end. Then, if they do not follow, walk away.

Understand that you cannot fix an abusive person. Abusive people are choosing to be abusive. The only way that they will change is if they choose to change. You will not be able to force them into changing or help them change. Do not change yourself to appease them into changing as it will never work.

Do not blame yourself. You may hear that everything is your fault, and you might even begin to think that it is, but remember, that is the manipulation. It is not your fault that someone else chooses to do something.

Do not engage with an abusive person. This is difficult...like, really, really difficult. When someone is hovering over you saying that you do things that you would never do, it is near impossible to not reply. However, whether in person or via text message, train your mind to focus on something else at the time. Maybe sing a little song in your head, count to ten, turn the phone off if they will not stop texting, text yourself the responses instead, write down how you would respond, or get up and walk away.

Work on creating an exit plan. We all picture what life would be like outside of the reigns of an abuser. Why not create that on paper and try to set up a way to make that happen? Yes, it is very scary, and you may not follow through with it, but sometimes all it takes is writing out what you wish to do. During this time, it would be best to meet with a domestic violence advocate or a counselor to assist with coming up with a proper plan.

You may also notice that you are developing unhealthy coping mechanisms in order to deal with your situation. Some might start drinking alcohol, eating fatty foods, stop exercising, start laying in bed a lot, begin drinking soda or pop, and/or not eating at all. There are plenty of other bad coping mechanisms, but either way, it is a way to take your mind off of the chaos around you to give you a sense of control as well as a bit of happiness as you indulge.

Recognizing signs of abuse is one thing, but what do you do if you are experiencing it? Well, if you find yourself in this situation and do not think you have a way out—which is very common—to ease your mind you can create a safety plan. A safety plan could include:

1. Keeping a suitcase at a neighbor's house,

2. Getting a folding ladder to keep in a room upstairs so you can escape,

3. Parking in the driveway and not in the garage,

4. Barricading yourself in a room with a heavy object, and

5. Giving a trusted friend or family member a key or garage door opener to your home.

There are other ways to escape; however, if you are living in an abusive situation, but these are the first steps to take in order to safely get out of the home. When all other options fail, protect yourself and your children, if you have any.

Chapter 11

----- ❧❦❧ -----

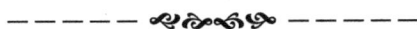

How to Heal from Narcissistic Abuse

When you are attempting to heal from the narcissist after escaping, somewhere during the determination stage, you will need to find ways to take care of yourself. You need to heal all of the wounds that the narcissist's abuse left behind in order to become the person you are meant to be. Healing can be incredibly difficult if left to your own devices, and you may even feel tempted to move on without ever addressing the harm you endured. However, it is essential. You will never truly heal if you leave the wounds to fester and worsen. Your sense of self, your happiness, and you, yourself, will slowly wither away if you do not treat the wounds. Just as you know, you must treat a physical wound; you must care for your mental and emotional wounds as well. Take the time to really absorb the methods of healing from abuse, and really put effort into bettering yourself. You will feel so much relief after you have taken the time to heal.

Remember, running away or putting your head in the sand and pretending that you are fine is what the narcissist taught you to do. No matter how tempting it may be to try to grit your teeth and move on, you need to address your injuries. In moments of weakness, remind yourself that you only want to do what is familiar, but doing so will not help or benefit you. It is simply falling back to old ways that can lead to a further setback, and potentially send you spiraling back to the narcissist. Only by healing all of the wounds can you truly remove all of the chains the narcissist has installed and really free yourself.

Self-Care

One of the easiest ways, in theory, to help heal yourself is to engage in self-care. Self-care can be difficult for even those with healthy minds, who are happy with themselves and do not have some serious healing to do. It is easy to get caught up in the bustle of life and give up the self-care time in favor of doing something else, but it is important to engage in.

Self-care, at its core, is taking care of yourself. You are making your physical and mental wellbeing a priority for yourself, and you are not ashamed of doing so. Particularly for the victims of narcissistic abuse, who have internalized that their needs are met last, this can be difficult, but it is an important skill to learn. The easiest way to engage in self-care is to create a routine in which you have several things that you do regularly in order to create good habits. If you are unsure where to start with self-care, here are several ideas of ways to start your self-care routine.

- Good sleep hygiene: Make sure you are going to sleep at the same time every night and pay attention to things that could make sleeping difficult, such as having a television in your room that keeps you awake or using your phone in the dark in bed. Keep the bedroom just for sleep!

- Eat healthy food: Make it a point to nourish your body to keep it physically healthy. Your gut and your mind are believed to be linked, and if you can keep your gut healthy, you will likely find your mental health improvements as well.

- Exercise daily: Exercise is not just good for the body —the mind needs it as well. Make it a point to take at least thirty minutes a day to exercise, whether it is a fitness class, time at the gym, or even just a stroll through the park. Just make sure that stroll gets your heart rate up!

- Prioritize self-care: The easiest way to engage in self-care is to prioritize self-care. Make sure that you guard the times you set aside for caring for yourself and treat them as precious. You deserve that time for your own well-being.

- Take a trip: Sometimes, taking a weekend vacation away from the bustle of work, friends, and the city can be incredibly refreshing. This works even better if you disconnect for a while and just let yourself enjoy your own presence. Keep your phone off, and enjoy your own company for a bit!

- Take breaks often: Mental health breaks are necessary to function effectively. Without them, you risk burning out and otherwise struggling to meet your responsibilities without being utterly miserable. Your breaks could even be simple five-minute breaks outside every couple of hours when working. Your sanity will definitely thank you for it.

- Caring for a pet: Pets bring an awful lot to our lives, even with the responsibilities that come with them. By having a pet, you encourage a relationship with something that is unconditional, lacking judgment, and can even lower your blood pressure. Dogs, in particular, are so good for self-care and healing that even PTSD sufferers have adapted them as service animals to help with mental health!

- Staying organized: If you are organized, you are less likely to stress out about forgetting something or how to fit everything in. Even something as simple as implementing a calendar or planner can benefit your mental health immensely.

- Cook at home: Along with eating healthily, cooking your own food can be surprisingly therapeutic. There is just something about taking raw ingredients, preparing them, and creating something nourishing and delicious from them that is so satisfying! Cook at home often to reap the benefits.

- Read: Read often. Not only is it good for your brain, but there is also a world of knowledge out there. You could even read a book about learning self-care! Even if the books you read are fiction, you can still benefit from reading. It keeps your mind stimulated and will help keep you healthier.

- Learn a new skill: Learning something new can help you raise your own self-esteem. At finally learning to do something new, you are likely to feel proud of yourself, which is great! Try learning something new, especially if it is something that has always interested you.

Compassion

As there is even an entire stage in the healing process called compassion, it comes as no surprise that it plays a part in healing from your abuse. Remember to have the compassion for yourself to acknowledge that you did not deserve the abuse you endured, and to recognize that making mistakes is okay.

Oftentimes, victims of narcissistic abuse struggle to be compassionate or patient with themselves—they feel as though they are underserving of that compassion, even if they would tell anyone else in their shoes that it is okay and that compassion is necessary. Even little things can set off a victim of abuse, such as spilling a glass of milk. If you have endured abuse, you may tell yourself that you are stupid for making such a simple mistake, and you may even belittle yourself, calling yourself a klutz and worthless.

The problem is, those are not your words—they are the narcissists. Spilling a glass of milk is not a big deal in the grand scheme of things. In terms of a mistake, it is harmless. Even if the glass shattered, no one died. There was no irreparable damage to anything other than a glass, that most likely does not have some immense value anyway.

Remember to regard yourself with the same compassion you have always had for others. You deserve it just as much as the people you treat with that compassion and directing some of that inward does not take away from anyone else either. The compassion and willingness to forgive yourself will go a long way.

That compassion should also come with patience. Recognize that it will take a significant amount of time for yourself to heal from the narcissist's abuse, but that does not invalidate you. That does not make you less valuable, and it does not say anything about your worth. It simply means that you are a human and you are likely to have roadblocks from time to time. Just because you trip and fall and make a mistake does not mean you should berate yourself or make yourself feel worse.

Allow Yourself Time to Grieve Properly

Grief is a natural part of living, in which people cope with loss. Typically, grief is reserved for people who have lost a close family member or friend, but as you go through the stages of separating yourself from an abusive relationship, you go through a similar process. This is because, particularly when involved with a narcissist, you have lost someone. You have lost the person you thought the narcissist was. Remember how the narcissist used a persona to draw you in—you fell in love with the narcissist's mask. You initially loved someone who turned out to be a figment of your abuser's imagination. However, the process of watching the narcissist morph from a perfect lover into a monster is devastating. It is not unlike watching someone fade away from a terminal illness, slowly losing him—but when you lose the narcissist's persona, you are left with a monster wearing your loved one's face as a constant reminder of what you lost.

When you met the narcissist for the first time, you saw someone charming, charismatic, friendly, and likely every single thing you have ever wanted. You essentially saw your soulmate standing in front of you, and over time, your soulmate faded away. First, the person you trusted with everything started to hurt you, a little at first, until the abuse was nearly constant. You were left, dismayed how someone you loved so deeply, who you thought loved you just as passionately, could suddenly shift into a monster, but he did. This is just as profound of a loss, even if you are losing the idea of a person. You still lost someone that you loved, and you should not minimize that. Grief comes in five stages: denial, anger, bargaining, depression, and acceptance.

Denial

When you get to denial, you want to deny that anything has happened. This was when you were ensnared by the narcissist, entirely convinced that the abuse was not as bad as it actually was. You denied that the person you loved was gone. After all, how could he be gone when you can see his face right there? You hold onto hope that the person you thought the narcissist was is still in there somewhere, and you make excuses. You may say that the narcissist was not so bad, or try to convince yourself that you are willing to stay behind because at least you get to see your loved one's face looking back at you through the abuse. You attempt to convince yourself that things will be okay. This is where you were before you reached the acknowledgment stage of healing. You refused to recognize the abuse for what it was.

Anger

Eventually, your denial gives in to anger. Your eyes are opened, and you finally want to break free. At this stage, you want to escape at all costs, telling yourself that you do not deserve this abuse. You feel angry at the narcissist for convincing you to stay with him, and for convincing you that the abuse is acceptable or normal. You feel angry that the person you loved is gone, or never existed in the first place. You feel betrayed and manipulated—because you were. The narcissist played a dirty trick on you, and you fell for it. More than anything, though, you feel angry at yourself for falling for it all. You tell yourself that you should have known better and you also push the blame onto yourself, even if you do not deserve it. You desperately want for the person you love to come back somehow, and you want the narcissist to pay for what he did to you. This is likely the stage in which you flee from the narcissist's abuse, no longer willing to put up with it anymore.

Bargaining

When you reach the bargaining stage, you are willing to give anything to return to the way things were before. You tell yourself that you will do whatever it takes to have the narcissist's persona back, whether it is putting up with the narcissist's abuse or anything else. At this stage, you are grappling with the permanence of the situation and are desperate for a sign that reality is not what it may seem. If you are religious, you may pray to your god to fix things, or that you will be more devout if your god can somehow give you a miracle and bring your loved one back to you without the narcissist. You promise to do anything that comes to mind, but of course, it does not work because your loved one was never a real, living person.

Depression

Soon after, you come to the realization of the permanence of the current situation. You see that you will never get your love back, and you fall into a depression. You are beside yourself that the person is gone and you are so miserable and unhappy with it that you stop feeling anything at all. You essentially turn off your feelings, instead of staying in self-pity. You recognize the futility of it all and wonder why you should even bother continuing with anything. Life feels hopeless, and you wonder if even the narcissist would be a better alternative than this hell alone. You miss the narcissist's persona so much it hurts, and the idea of never seeing that person you loved again is so overwhelming that you struggle to cope.

Acceptance

Eventually, you finally reach the stage of acceptance. Here, you finally see the light again. You recognize that the narcissist tricked you, but you also recognize that things will be okay. You still love the persona that you originally fell for, but you recognize that he was nothing but an attempt to manipulate you into falling for the narcissist. You see it for the weapon it was, and you accept letting it go. At this point, you seek to move forward, and you allow yourself to find enjoyment in other things and realize that what happened was not the end of the world and that you are open to the idea of finding real love again in the future.

Develop Support Networks

Recognizing that you cannot get through this process alone is probably one of the most indicative of whether you will be able to escape the narcissist's abuse. You need the support of other people to be there for you in moments of weakness, and when you feel like you can no longer go on without the narcissist. Having people, you can talk to and trust to help guide you makes you far more likely to make it through without going back to the narcissist for further abuse. Your support network can take many forms, but most of the time, it is built upon a foundation of four groups of people: Friends, family, support groups, and a therapist, if you have one.

Friends

Friends will be there for you through thick and thin, and even if the narcissist has managed to isolate you from many of them, if you were to send a message to some of your closest friends from before the abuse, you would likely be surprised about how many of them are relieved and thrilled to hear from you. They may share that they have been waiting for you to contact them for ages and that they were always so concerned for you. Your friends will likely make up the bulk of your support group. These are people who will meet up with you on a bad day to watch movies and binge eat cartons of ice cream, or will let you rant about just how betrayed you feel by the narcissist. They will gladly be there for you and simply enjoy being in your presence in general. If you do not have friends, you should try to make some. There are many different ways you can do so, such as going to classes to learn new skills or groups you can join with people who share your interests. Especially with the internet at your disposal, you can likely google any hobby of yours and the city you live in, and be surprised to find groups of like-minded individuals that would probably be thrilled to have you if you contacted them and asked to join.

Family

Your family will likely be there for you if you ask for more serious help, such as needing money, a place to stay, or general support while trying to escape. Especially if you are escaping with children, your own family is a fantastic place to start. Your family only wants what is best for you, and as your friends, you may be surprised to hear that many of your family members had suspected abuse for a long time. They will also likely be relieved at you leaving, and you can frequently find plenty of support from these people.

Support groups

Support groups are particularly useful when you need someone that understands what you are going through more so than just having a general idea of how you felt. You can typically find support groups for narcissistic abuse survivors by searching online, both in your own area and online. There are several different forums and boards of people who get together to discuss their abuse, and you will likely be able to find other people that have gone through almost exactly what you have. The people that will understand the intensity of the abuse, the way the narcissist so thoroughly manages to break people down, and how hard it is to leave are the ones who have gone through it before and know it out of the experience.

When you find a support group that clicks for you, you will be able to see people at all stages of healing. You will see people who have more or less fully recovered and are there, supporting other people through their journeys toward healing, and others who may have just left, or have been considering leaving that are trying to learn what to do. This can be particularly useful, as you can look at other people who are further along than you are for inspiration. You can ask for advice, talk to people who have been where you are, and even just enjoy a conversation with someone who knows what you have gone through. Ultimately, this can be an incredibly insightful experience, and you will almost always get something good out of browsing through these forums or meeting up with other survivors. What will be clear when you do this, however, is that you are not alone by any means. Many, many people have fallen victim to the narcissist, and unfortunately, many more will as well. At the very least, there are several safe spaces on the internet and in person where the survivors of narcissistic abuse can come together to support each other toward healing and bettering themselves.

Therapist

A therapist can be particularly useful in helping heal as well. While you will have a professional relationship with a therapist as opposed to a friendship, you will be able to talk to the therapist to help you deal with difficult feelings or to deal with things that you are struggling to handle. The therapist, though optional, is always a fantastic choice when recovering from abuse if you can make it happen.

Creating Healthy Outlets

When you have suffered through narcissistic abuse, you have probably developed some pretty toxic thoughts and feelings yourself. Many of these come from what is likely a tendency toward being empathetic, as that is one of the things the narcissist desires most, and you absorbed the narcissist's toxic feelings. Empaths are particularly prone to internalizing the feelings and tendencies of those around them, and the tendencies of the narcissist can be particularly toxic to the empath.

One of the best things to do when you have internalized all of that negativity is finding a creative, healthy outlet for it. You should seek out some sort of way to eliminate the toxicity from you, whether through art, music, learning, taking classes, or anything else that appeals to you. Exercising is a common tactic used, in which you literally sweat out the negativity. The important part here is that you manage to eliminate it in some way and that you feel better after you have finished whatever you have chosen to do. Over time, you will release all of the pent-up negativity, and you will begin to feel much better about yourself.

Therapy

Therapy can guide you toward healing as well. As briefly touched upon, a therapist is one of the greatest favors you can do for yourself. There are very few people in this world who would not benefit from therapy, and the likelihood of one of them being you is incredibly slim. The sooner you start it, the sooner you will start seeing results. There are several different kinds of therapy that could be useful for a victim of narcissistic abuse, and through therapy, you would be able to learn valuable skills, such as how to cope with the trauma left behind, understanding what made you vulnerable to the narcissist in the first place, and how to solve all of the problems that come with all of the emotions you feel whirling around within you.

If therapy is something that sounds like it would benefit you, try speaking to your primary care doctor for a referral, or seek out recommendations local to your area online. Even if the cost is an issue, there are plenty that will help you on a sliding scale, as well as online options that may be more affordable for you.

Conclusion

————— ❧ ⊰⊱ ❧ —————

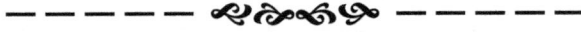

This book is not meant to prevent any harm from befalling you. Abuse is scary and the people behind it are unpredictable. It can be terrifying to try to deal with abusers head-on, and you are incredibly brave for doing so. If nothing else, appreciate yourself and your bravery already for being able to keep calm in the midst of a potentially dangerous relationship.

You are someone who can deal with anything if you can deal with an abuser or a toxic relationship. If you can look an abuser in the eye and know that someday, you'll be far away from them, that's more empowering than anything. The day I left my abuser was perhaps the scariest day I ever experienced throughout the entirety of the relationship. My blood ran cold, and I had no idea if they would find me and what they would do if they did. It's so empowering to be able to deal with the trials of abuse while still thinking about what you'll do after you make it out. Your abuser is cold and manipulative, and they will do anything they can to make it so that you never leave. This is their ultimate goal—keep their prey around for as long as possible until they've used up every ounce of spirit in their victim.

Despite this, you have many tools at your disposal to make use of your strengths when you do figure it out. After you address your weaknesses along with your strengths, you can figure out what to do from there based on what your particular situation calls for. That's also where this book comes in handy—there are countless different types of abuse and many different ways that abuse can manifest. Therefore, there are also countless different ways that you can react to that abuse properly and defend yourself against it.

This book is not only to determine how you're being abused and how you can keep yourself from falling for those tricks, but it's also to get you to consider where to go from there. Many books on abuse don't properly take into account the unpredictability of life immediately after a volatile relationship. Being able to look for different ways out, make notes of your abuser's behavior, and have different escape plans available can save you a trouble when you finally make your escape.

If you feel that this book has helped to empower you to grow past your abuse and take matters safely into your own hands,

I'd be delighted if you would leave a review to let other people know your story and that they are not alone.